AF383158

SHY RADICALS

جذريون خجولون

SHY RADICALS

جذريون خجولون

THE ANTISYSTEMIC POLITICS OF THE MILITANT INTROVERT

HAMJA AHSAN

CONTENTS

ACKNOWLEDGEMENTS
HAMJA AHSAN

This book is written on the back of a lifetime of resentment.

I am on a never-ending world tour to overthrow extrovert-supremacy. Follow @shyradicals Please support: patreon.com/hamja. Your support saves me from destitution.

'The Shy Radicals' (2020) film is directed by Tom Dream, produced by Black Dog Films, and funded by BFI. Screenings: #ShyRadicalsFilm.

I would like to thank Nina Power for her kindness and for her belief in the Shy Radicals cause, which kept my head above water at the lowest of times.

Thank you to the many people whose life experiences of oppression reminded me why I needed to write this book. Post #ShyPower salutes. Vote #VoteAspergistan.

A quiet whisper to Nicholas Brown, formerly at the Stuart Hall Library (the best of Sensitive White Men) and Alexandra Phillips, Mira Hammad, Kealoha Umika for their help on the final manuscripts.

The book continues to inspire a global trail of fan-made art works the world over: #introfada

I am influenced by my favourite radio show podcasts, 'Law and Disorder' and 'Political Prisoner Radio'.

I acknowledge the model of Barnor Hesse's 'Eight White Identities' as the model for Extrovert Identities.

I take inspiration from the solicitor Gareth Peirce (who represented and advocated for my brother Talha), whose subdued manner of speaking, humility and media shyness I always took to be proto-Shy Radical.

I dedicate this book to the Shy Radical struggle.

Any resemblance of any character to anyone fictitious or real, living or dead, is purely coincidental, as every character in this book is entirely based on myself.

Not so very long ago, the earth numbered 7 billion inhabitants: 6 billion were quiet unassuming types, and the other billion domineering, colonising bores. The former had the Word, but chose to speak it very quietly, the others just shouted and pushed people over until they got their way. The loud elite sought to manufacture a native loudness – they picked out quiet teenagers, taking them from their bedrooms, they branded them, as if with a nightclub-stamp, with the principles of extrovert culture. But these fake loud-people had nothing to say to their quiet brothers and sisters, they could only echo the beats they longed to escape from.

Then the quiet ones began to speak, but it was not speech as we loud ones understood. In fact, we couldn't understand it at all. What? Were they able to be quiet *on their own terms*? But surely they owe the very power of silence to those who had taught it to them while shrieking and laughing like hyenas! We were upset that they had not accepted our ideals. Amongst ourselves we still laughed at them, those quiet ones, 'Let them be silent, it relieves their feelings; hedgehogs that whisper can surely not organise any kind of revolt against us.'

Many of these early 'Shy Radicals', the patient ones, tried to explain what we had done to them, and how their lives did not hang together in the Loud World. What they were claiming was this: 'You have forced us to speak; your *loudism* claims we are at one with the rest of loud society but your punishment of shy peoples sets us apart.' Pretending we couldn't hear them, we pretended to listen: administrators of hedonism are not paid to read Hegel, or indeed anything at all. When we closed the libraries we did not listen to them; when we sold off the forests and quiet gardens, we refused to read their beautifully-written petitions. We even offered some of them prizes, or gave them 'quiet rooms' at universities, even though we refused to cut the radio or ban noisy people from these spaces.

2017. Listen: 'Let us waste no time in whispered accusations and uncomfortable pretence. Leave these loud continents where they are never done talking, and forcing everyone else to talk, and killing us with their volume while pretending to understand the struggle of the quiet person.' The tone is new. Who dares to speak thus? It is a Shy Radical, a person from the Quiet World. When we discovered the writings set out before you, these documents of a place called Aspergistan, following a quiet revolution (the so-called 'Introfada'), we were astonished. And if you shout, pained, that 'They are going to force us all to shut-up!' the true nature of reality escapes you; for the Shy Radicals has nothing in it for you at all. In short, the Quiet World finds itself and whispers to itself in its own voice. We struggle to hear it because we are not used to listening, only to the constant jammer of our own violent self-congratulation, at art openings, house parties, pubs and every place where the quiet person is oppressed. And we do not notice.

Thus there is a fresh moment of quietness; and this time we ourselves are involved, for by its nature quietness is changing us. Every one of us must be quiet for him or herself – and quiet therefore for all. This book has not the slightest need for a preface, all the less because it is not addressed to us. Yet I have written one, in order to bring the argument to its conclusion; for we in the Loud World too are being *deshoutified*: that is to say that the shouty-person that is in every one of us is being savagely rooted out. Let us listen to ourselves, if we can pause for one second, and hear what is becoming of us. We must face that unexpected revelation, the uncovering of our loudism. There you can hear it, quite unnecessarily booming, and it's not a pretty sound. It was nothing but an ideology of sound-lies, a perfect justification for the oppression of shy peoples; its decibels, its recourse to hedonism and 'fun' were only alibis for our aggressions.

ONE

DRAFT CONSTITUTION OF
THE SHY PEOPLE'S REPUBLIC
OF ASPERGISTAN

SHY PEOPLE'S REPUBLIC OF ASPERGISTAN

WE, THE PEOPLES OF ASPERGISTAN,

EMBODY THE SHY PEOPLE'S REPUBLIC OF ASPERGISTAN – the sanctuary, beacon and homeland of oppressed Shy, Introvert and Autistic Spectrum peoples – and understand that our nation's crowning principles will serve as a bulwark against the hegemony of the Extrovert World Order, marking a decisive step toward the fraternal and sororal collaboration and co-existence of all Shy Peoples in an autonomous worldwide union.

ACKNOWLEDGE that successive generations of our people have suffered rejection, bullying, humiliation, belittlement, pathologisation, persecution, subjugation, exploitation, erasure, exclusion, alienation, discrimination and disadvantage at the hands of the global system of Extrovert-Supremacism, which has dispossessed and deprived us of our right to introspective life, self-esteem, equality and peace.

DEMAND the reversal of the operations of Extrovert-exclusive representation in congress and debate-chamber parliaments, acknowledging the system's failure to listen to and represent its subjects and citizens. We take Lao Tzu's dictum 'the quieter you become, the more you are able to hear' as the foundational principle of our democratic institutions.

CHERISH the richness of inner life – silence, contemplation, reflective solitude, intimate company, investigative depths, peer-reviewed truth – which forms the basis and legitimacy of the state and government to determine our destiny.

PROSPECTIVE TERRITORIES

Acknowledging the failure of the 1947 partition of the Indian subcontinent, territories will consist of a third, shy identity-based partition. The new partition will question the basis on which the land was originally divided according to a now defunct identity politics of religious identity, which we seek to replace with a new identity politics relating to introvert life. The proposed shy partition will consist of territories formerly known as:

1. *North-West Frontier Province of Pakistan and semi autonomous regions.*
2. *The caves and mountainous regions of Afghanistan, excluding Kabul.*
3. *The Islamic republic of Iran, excluding Tehran.*

These territories will be united into a single federal state at the centre of Aspergistan. The capital of the state will be Qom – the city of religious scholars.

Parliament may by law add further states to the federation.
All territories are to be governed by the Shyria legislative system.
No extradition treaty will be signed with any external territory or nation-state.

CHAPTER 1

FUNDAMENTAL POLITICS

ARTICLE 1.

The Shy People's Republic of Aspergistan is an independent Pan-Shyist state representing the interests of all Shy, Introvert and Autistic Spectrum peoples, herein referred to as Aspergistan.

ARTICLE 2.

Aspergistan is a revolutionary vanguard state guided by anti-systemic Introvert ideology, which constitutes the world outlook and political foundation of the state.

ARTICLE 3.

Aspergistan honours the struggle of the Introfada in the liberation of the homeland and the freedom, tranquillity and well-being of the Shy Peoples within and without its sovereign territory.

ARTICLE 4.

Aspergistan shall champion the rights of Shy People overseas, as defined by International Shyria Law, and provide diplomatic and emotional support.

ARTICLE 5.

Aspergistan shall reinforce international cooperation and maintain friendly diplomatic relations with subjects and bodies within nations committed to the safeguarding of Introvert Spectrum culture.

A R T I C L E 6.

Aspergistan shall pursue a separatist path of development – independent of Popular Girl approval – against all hierarchical imitation of the Extrovert-Supremacist world camp. Aspergistan shall neither compete, nor cooperate, with the Enemy.

A R T I C L E 7.

The Shy, Introvert and Autistic Spectrum Peoples represent a united front that will permanently resist divide and rule tactics. Our unity is based on our collective experiences of bullying and humiliation within the Extrovert-ruled world.

A R T I C L E 8.

Mainstream life has no place in Aspergistan. All politics will remain underground.

A R T I C L E 9.

Civic privilege will only be granted to the voice of the unheard.

CHAPTER 2

THE STRUCTURE OF THE STATE

ARTICLE 10.

All central and local power belongs to the Shy Peoples. No position of government or parliamentary representation shall be held by the Extrovert-class or by their collaborators.

ARTICLE 11.

Any declarations, resolutions and motions made on a stage or raised platform will be seen to not represent the people.

ARTICLE 12.

Any past declarations, resolutions and motions made on a stage or raised platform will be regarded as void and illegitimate.

ARTICLE 13.

All politics of distraction, media soundbites, and the pictorial representation of election candidates prior to election will be abolished.

ARTICLE 14.

A thoroughly referenced and peer-reviewed guide to the policy proposals of each of the electoral candidates is to be to be scattered on the shores of national beaches and on park benches, non-invasively encouraging all citizens to independently research electoral choices in their own time.

ARTICLE 15.

Abolition of debate chamber and vocal debate processes as the primary site of legislative representation and decision making. All legislative decisions will be arrived at following solitary contemplation by the executive, at a time and location determined by Shyria law judges.

ARTICLE 16.

The state may not alert its presence to its citizens by means of noise. The prohibition of noise-based alerts will extend to sirens, alarm bells and emergency calls. The state guarantees the right to silence before all law enforcement organs.

CHAPTER 3

FUNDAMENTAL RIGHTS AND DUTIES OF CITIZENS

ARTICLE 17.

Introversion is inviolable. No person may disturb its peace or violate its freedom.

The state shall guarantee: freedom from small talk; freedom from coercive visual distraction; freedom from enforced jollity or coerced happiness; freedom from Extrovert harassment during leisure time and national holidays; the right to stay in one's home during leisure time and national holidays; freedom from superficial judgement based on outward appearances and consumer choices; freedom from frivolous public media assaults; freedom from stigmatisation for the pursuit of an introvert life; freedom from Extrovert epistemic violence, including all accusations of being anti-social or aloof.

Disrupting the concentration of Aspergistan citizens will be taken seriously and punished in full accordance with the law.

ARTICLE 18.

No one shall be required to attend or perform at social gatherings.

ARTICLE 19.

The State grants special protection to children and young people, and bans the use of Extrovert-normative teen categories (such as 'nerd', 'jock', 'cool', 'geek', 'square', 'keener', 'weirdo', 'loner', 'loser', 'freak', 'dork', 'emo', 'dweeb'). In the interests of healthy development and the maintenance of self-esteem, it guarantees the absolute protection of quiet children against bullying, peer pressure and introvert hate crime.

ARTICLE 20.

The State guarantees support for the healing and recovery of all persons adversely affected by the pressure, damage and trauma exerted upon them by Extrovert-Supremacist states, Introvert Hate groups and Trendy Club.

CHAPTER 4

NATIONAL FLAG, NATIONAL ANTHEM, CULTURAL SYMBOL AND CAPITAL CITY

ARTICLE 21.

The Shy Radical state declares the following a charade and part of Extrovert Supremacist ideology from which Aspergistanis seek emancipation: Patriotic public ceremonies; Military parades; Jingoism; Celebration of state representatives; Shallow mythologising of historical conflicts and tragedies; Street parties and flashing firework displays.

ARTICLE 22.

The flag of Aspergistan consists of a black flag punctuated thusly '...' The ellipsis will be represented as three dark blue circles symbolising silence and the depths of the ocean. The flag will never be publicly hoisted. The flag may be used only by citizens wishing to silently indicate their request for quiet, solitude, and personal space. It will be the shared responsibility of citizens to respect the wishes of the flag bearer.

ARTICLE 23.

For sporting or cultural fixtures abroad, opposing or host countries will be required to listen to our national anthem using seashells. Aspergistan shall ensure the provision of a fit supply of seashells to the opposing team of the foreign representative nation. This listening shall be equal to the length of singing or public cheerleading displays by Extrovert-Supremacist states.

ARTICLE 24.

The national anthem is the sound of a seashell, which may be accessed on a twenty-four-hour-basis by citizens via the holding of the shell to the ear. Non-citizens outside the current territory of Aspergistan may also access the anthem in this manner.

ARTICLE 25.

No citizen or representative of the state of Aspergistan shall be obliged to sing the national anthem of any other state, whether at formal ceremonies or sporting occasions.

ARTICLE 26.

Aspergistan shall boycott any sporting or cultural event that does not accord with the above Articles.

ARTICLE 27.

Aspergistan will boycott any sporting or cultural event that does not ensure Autism-friendly facilities, or show due respect to the rights of Autistic Spectrum people.

ARTICLE 28.

Representing the rich life of the underground, the national flower will be represented by the roots of plants and trees, embedded in soil. Shy Radicals acknowledge the privileging of the blooming flower image to be part of the systemic enforcement of Extrovert normativity.

ARTICLE 29.

The first capital will be Qom in the first map of speculative territories, functioning as a city of scholars and seminarians. It forms the capital-in-exile whilst awaiting the Aspergistani revolution.

CHAPTER 5

CULTURE

———

ARTICLE 30.

Abolition of private views, opening ceremonies, launch parties and all other suffocating crowd-gathering forms of the celebration of new cultural products, film seasons and exhibitions. The state encourages the purging of the socialite-class.

ARTICLE 31.

The state shall safeguard and preserve all areas of solitary dwelling under public ownership from outside interference, e.g. caves, forests, mountains, rivers and woods. The state guarantees the right to clear and empty space in all spheres of life.

ARTICLE 32.

The state shall guarantee twenty-four-hour access to all public libraries, museums, laboratories, book shops, tea and coffee houses, archives and cathedrals within its sovereign territory.

ARTICLE 33.

The night culture of the state shall honour the sacred contemplative nature of the dark as a journey into the soul, a time of rest and exploration. Abolition of Trendy Club culture and its colonisation of t-time space will be guaranteed by the will of the unheard.

ARTICLE 34.

The state guarantees twenty-four-hour access to all objects of artistic, historical and cultural value.

ARTICLE 35.

Aspergistan will adopt a revolutionary system for the measurement of time, developing a new calendar based on Eastern Lunar models. This will abolish the concepts of the weekend, A.M. and P.M.

ARTICLE 36.

Aspergistan shall adopt its own internal units of measurement of distance to ensure the safeguarding of empty space.

ARTICLE 37.

Aspergistan shall adopt its own internal system of measuring noise levels in accordance with Shyria Law, with inviolable introvert rights at its centre.

ARTICLE 38.

April 2nd is to be known as Worldwide Autism Day, designated by United Nations General Assembly Resolution 62/139. This will be the first day of a week of national holidays.

ARTICLE 39.

Abolition of strobe lighting, flashing lights, neon lighting and advertisement billboards from all public space, ensuring the clearest possible view of the constellations.

ARTICLE 40.

The biodiversity of flora and fauna shall be celebrated on the basis of whole eco-systems and the richness of the soil, rather than the privileging of flamboyant birds and animals and temporary blooming flower spans. Culls of flamboyant birds and animals and temporary blooming flower spans. Culls of flamboyant birds

with Shyria Supreme Court rulings. The state will also rescue
and preserve introvert biodiversity, recognising the historical
domestic genocidal cull of badgers, bats and deer in Extrovert-
Supremacist states.

ARTICLE 41.

Animals are not entertainment. Extrovert-Supremacist abuse of
animals for the purpose of showmanship and narcissism is abso-
lutely prohibited whether in the form of circus acts, magic tricks
or cats on Facebook.

CHAPTER 6

NATIONAL DEFENCE

ARTICLE 42.

All national armed forces and all national defence personnel will bear a coat of arms bearing the words 'Do Not Disturb'.

ARTICLE 43.

The state recognises the Extrovert-Supremacist weapons of celebrity-distraction, compulsive consumerism, headline populism, the privileging of frivolity and systemic mass ignorance to be the discursive weapons of Warfare of the Enemy. The Shy Radical states will prepare all necessary steps to provide countermeasures in the event of attack.

ARTICLE 44.

The permanent task of the Shy Underground People's Resistance Army is the consolidation and protection of its territory and citizens. Armed Isolationist units will be dispatched to counter Extrovert imperialism and expansionism.

ARTICLE 45.

Aspergistan declares the full-scale abolition of bravado and machismo within the ranks of the army, and its imitation within the public life of the state, recognising the complicity of military machismo with the formation of introvert hate crime.

 ARTICLE 46.

Aspergistan is the homeland of the deployment of guerrilla and underground tactics, protecting anonymity and invisibility, via the Shy Underground Ninja Assassin wing.

ARTICLE 47.

Aspergistan seeks to protect itself from all Extrovert-cyber-imperialist incursions by use of garbo, our state-developed firewall.

CHAPTER 7

ECONOMY & LABOUR RIGHTS

ARTICLE 48.

Aspergistan will ensure economic justice, esteem and recognition for Introvert labour. The Shy Radicals movement recognises the historical invisibility, subjugation, exploitation and the devaluing of Introvert labour, which it seeks to reverse through a Shyria-compliant economy.

ARTICLE 49.

For the purposes of resolving the problem of the exploitation and alienation of Introvert labour for Extrovert ends, the state declares the right to seize and to place under state control any private property used in the service of Extrovert-Supremacy. This include nightclubs and shopping malls, fields and pastures used for raves, streets used for Extrovert-harassment.

ARTICLE 50.

The Shy Radical movement recognises that economic justice is impossible in a celebrity-centric, model-centric and presenter-centric system where 'outgoingness' reigns supreme. All uneven economic and distributive power based on mass distraction is to be abolished. Researchers and those involved in behind-the-scenes jobs will be back-paid in full for their unrecognised work.

ARTICLE 51.

All advertising to be abolished for the protection of the mental health of the people.

ARTICLE 52.

Introvert Employment Centres will be set up in territories outside of the Aspergistan borders. These charitable centres will support alienated citizens of Extrovert-Supremacist states and assist them in finding soothing employment.

ARTICLE 53.

The state guarantees full lifetime pay and protection for all those pursuing independent research.

ARTICLE 54.

Aspergistan holds true to the dictum of proto-Shy Radical Benedict Spinoza, that 'freedom is knowledge of necessity'. The Shyria Court system recognises that mindless environmental destruction and the corrosion of spiritual values accords with the culture of bragging and ostentatiousness, and that compulsive consumerism brings destruction and exhaustion of the world's resources in the pursuit of insatiable decadent Extrovert extravagance.

ARTICLE 55.

Citizens are free from all compulsory appearances of false happiness and coerced amiability within the workplace. Office parties and networking events are suppressed and curtailed by the will of the unheard.

ARTICLE 56.

The architecture of all places of employment must conform to the dictates of Shyria Law. Reflective surfaces, neon, strobe lighting and open-planning will be strictly forbidden.

Abolition of Extrovert-risk as embodied by boom and bust roller-coaster economies, market speculation, and inflated salaries. The state will promote employment alternatives to the city trade floor.

ARTICLE 58.

The state resists corporate melancholia in the form of the commodification of introvert icons, culture, life and all tragic human history.

CHAPTER 8

RIGHT OF ASYLUM, EXIT AND ENTRY

ARTICLE 59.

Foreigners may be guaranteed entry to the state, provided they abide by Shyria Law for the duration of their visit. Citizens of the Extrovert-Supremacist family of nations may only be granted visas for periods of research, solitude and extended concentration.

ARTICLE 60.

Entry is guaranteed for those seeking escape from the assault of mass distraction, triviality and frivolity.

ARTICLE 61.

Asylum is guaranteed for all those engaged in struggle and resistance as part of the Pan-Shyist ideology. Safe passage from Extrovert-Supremacist states to Aspergistan will be provided for all those suffering political persecution.

ARTICLE 62.

Aspergistan is a safe haven for all Shy, Introvert and Autistic Spectrum people everywhere.

TWO

#OCCUPYBEDROOM

The death of social media is the birth of asocial media...
A wave of withdrawal is reshaping the political landscape...
Tremors can be felt from the global Shy Underground...
From the boardroom to the bedroom...

BREAKING TWEETS FROM THE #INTROFADA:
#OCCUPYBEDROOM #SILENTSTRIKE #BRINGBACKOURLIBRARIES
#FREEAMYLITTLEWOOD #INTROINTERVENTION #SHYSPRING
#INTROFADAASIA #INTROFADAEUROPE #INTROFADAAMERICAS
#ASPERGISTANNOW #PASSIVEINSURRECTION
#ALLPOWER2SHYPEOPLES #HIKIKOMORIWAVE

A Message from the Hikikomori Delegation (Tokyo, Japan)

[Translated in real-time from the Japanese by an International Shy Radical delegation]

WE ARE WITNESSING A NEW ERA OF REVOLT... #OCCUPYBEDROOM

For the Japanese Government, we are simply a social problem. For our families, we are parasites, or at best a cause for concern. An entire industry was brought into being to 'cure' us. But the Shy Radicals movement made us conscious. We don't need a cure: we are the vanguard revolt at the heart of advanced post-industrial capitalist society, and we are at the heart of the bourgeois home itself. We are not workers, not factory floor agitators; we are an inter-intervention, a passive insurrection from within the aspirational class...

The Japanese Government officially reckons that there are a million of us *hikikomori* peoples. But we cannot be quantified. The Ministry of Health define us as a negative social phenomenon. The official diagnosis comes once we have spent more than six months on strike in our bedrooms. We establish our picket lines as teenagers: studies underestimate our adolescent contingent when they say that we are mostly in our mid-twenties to early thirties. It is reported that we are 90% male and middle-class. But we defy all existing models of class struggle, just as we defy all recommended paths to 'adult' development. The government wants so-called therapists, counsellors, even Christian missionaries to make home visits to reintegrate us into mainstream society. We will not be integrated.

Why is the global news media so attentive to the stay-at-home lifestyle it persists in describing as 'dull'? Every global news agency has produced its own two-bit take, sometimes depicting traitor-*hikikomori* who will pander to some Orientalist picture of Japanese quiet society. It is said that we are non–communicative, yet our message has been making international news.

Most labour struggles would envy the amount of attention our strike is drawing. And our silence and reclusiveness means that our message cannot be misused or instrumentalised. We cannot be stopped.

We turned the world of aspiration on its head and we turned the regulatory working day inside out. Some of us, as an autonomous action, would sleep during office hours and stay awake during 'leisure hours'. There were too many 'successful' people in the world and they were bringing the world to ruin.

News is that *hikikomori* culture is catching on in South Korea. We are stopping the wave of the *Hallyu*: the wave of South Korean glossy pop culture.

People relate to us across borders. You cannot stop such international relations when they're made of nothing but mutual respect and solidarity against the generalised state of extroversion. Cases have been reported in Italy too. Society will eventually be brought to a standstill by our silent resistance. The resistance is fertile despite its stillness: we draw on a rich revolutionary history, inspired by other revolutionary bedroom cells and prison hunger strikes from Bobby Sands to Guantanamo Bay and the Short Corridor Collective of California Pelican Bay. We are at a new crossroads...

This *hikikomori* statement comes from a bedroom.

#OCCUPYBEDROOM

THREE

NEW LEXICON OF DEMOCRACY

The language of political communication is evolving.

As an organic development of the Introfada, a new democratic language is improvised as novel forms of representation are sought. All democratic decisions and motions are to be negotiated via a series of hand and body gestures to arrive at a consensus. Whilst previous non-hierarchical social movements had experimented with moving beyond the language of applause and booing with what we call 'wiggly hands' (also known by them as 'up twinkles' or 'spirit fingers'), the Shy Radicals movements nevertheless identify 'wiggly hands' as representing a serious democratic deficit.

This is a new dawn, a breath of fresh air... in the new century there will be no more rhetorical arm gestures at the podium...

A list of these communications were unfortunately handed to the 'anti-extremist' think-tank Vegas Foundation who integrated the lexicon into a government report as indications of potential radicalisation.

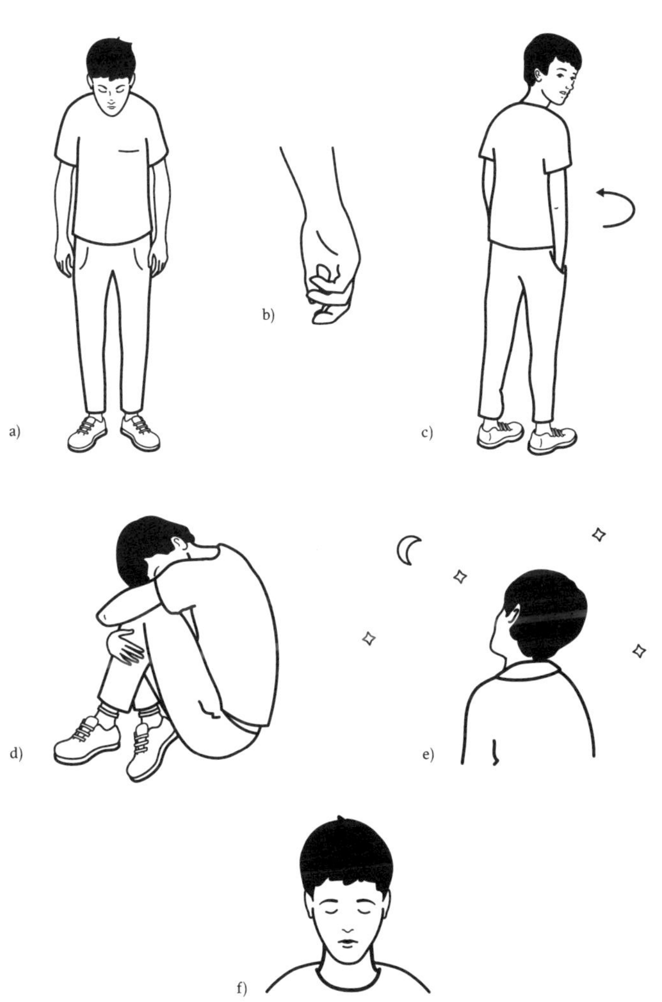

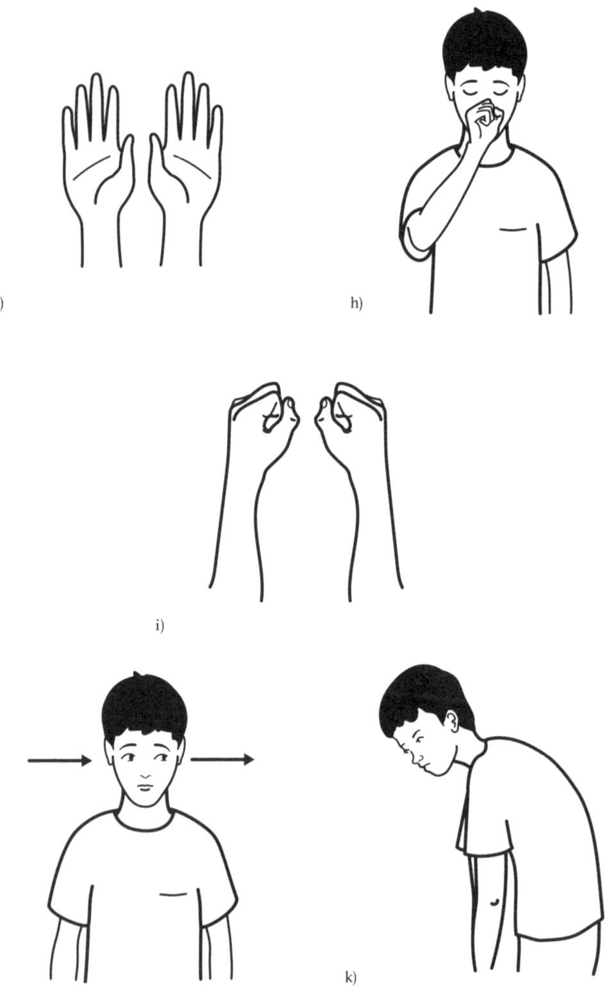

g)
h)
i)
j)
k)

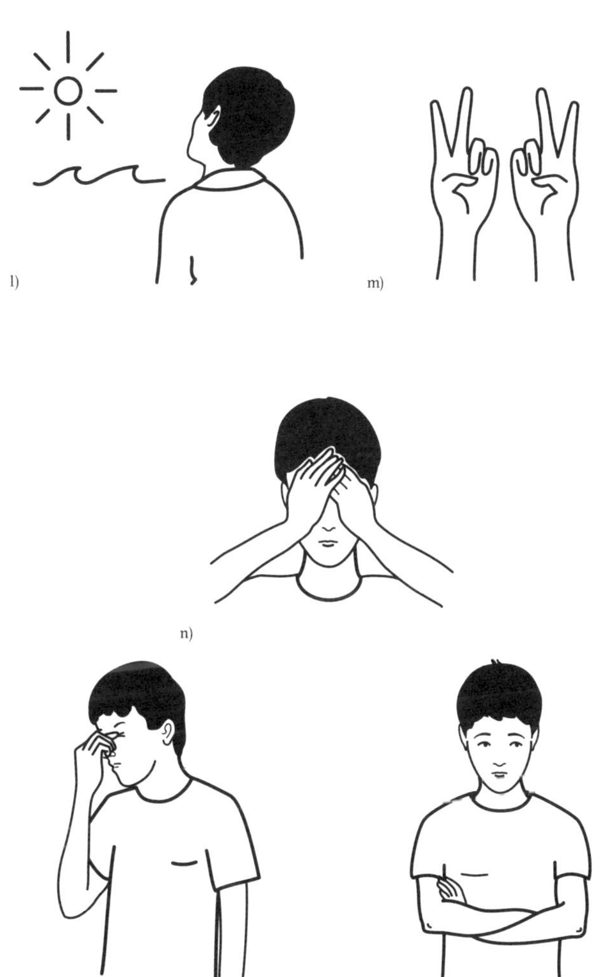

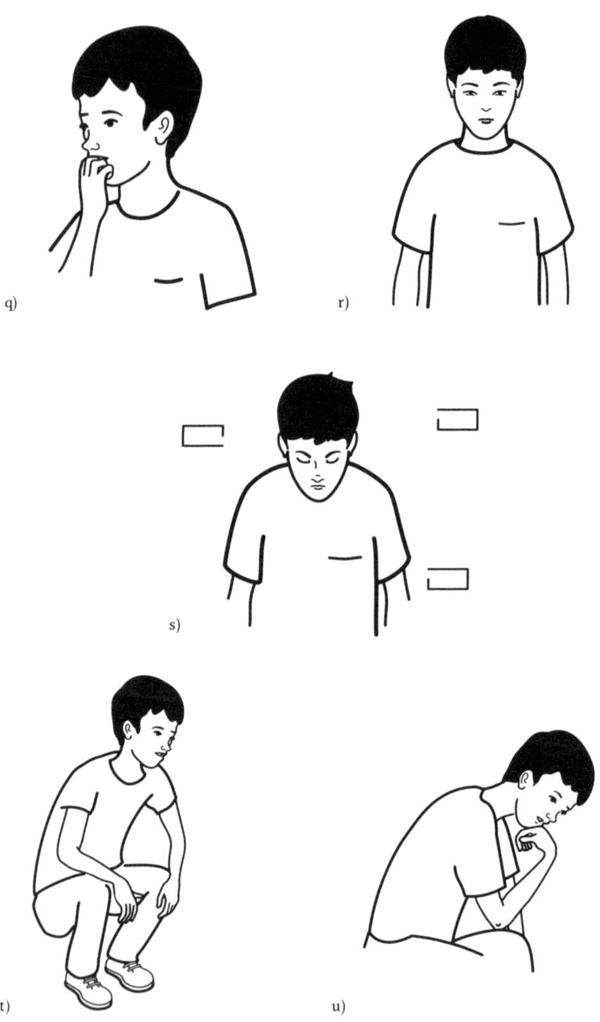

q)

r)

s)

t)

u)

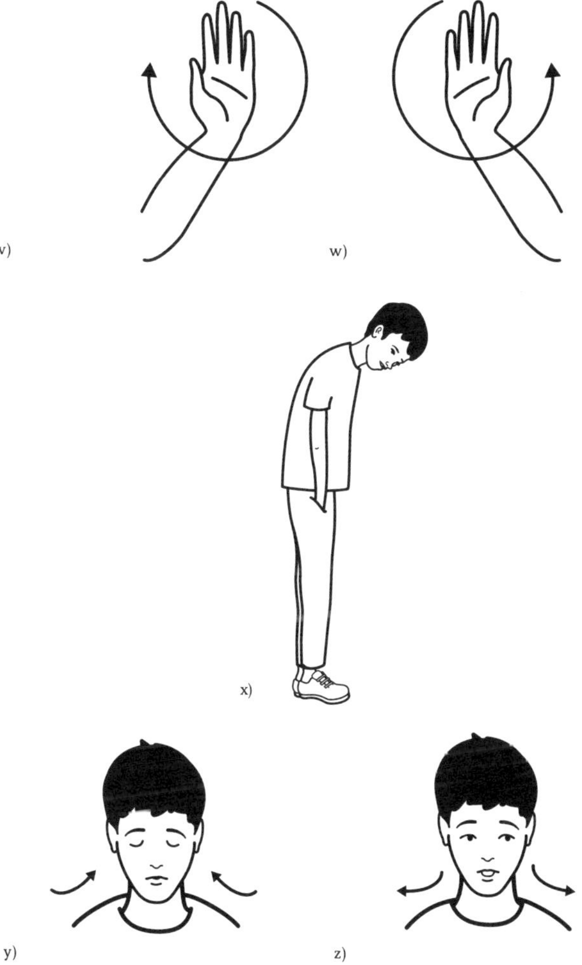

v)

w)

x)

y)

z)

a) staring at the floor
b) droop hands to the side
c) turning back
d) curling up on the floor
e) staring up at the sky
f) sighing
g) palms to open a book
h) curling fist in front of mouth
i) rock hand
j) averting eyes
k) hunchback
l) staring at the sea
m) scissorhands
n) running palms over face
o) rubbing eyes
p) arms folded
q) biting nails
r) squinting eyes
s) standing by wall
t) gathering around a fire
u) Rodin position
v) wax on
w) wax off
x) slouching
y) deep breath in
z) deep breath out

FOUR

PUBLIC STATEMENT: SHY RADICALS IS NOT A TERRORIST ORGANISATION

Shy Radicals is not a terrorist organisation...

Terrorism is always loud.

Guerrilla warfare was invented to make the business of conflict less noisy, less visible and less distracting. *Be among the people, as a fish in water.* Terrorism is to be distinguished from resistance, as terrorism is always very noisy. Explosions. Destruction of buildings. Gunfire. Hijackings. Terrorism, whether committed by states or by lone insurgents, is in each and every case Extrovert-Supremacist.

Terrorism and Extrovert-Supremacism exist on the same plane. Terrorism aspires to be the centre of attention. Attention is the central category of politics in Extrovert ideology. Attention is both the means and the ends. Attention without substance. Attention without merit. Attention without principle. Seeking attention in and of itself. This is the main motive of terrorist action. When the highest political leglisative and executive authority today cave in to the powers of distractive mass-media populism, terrorism seems like the only effective option in such a system. The system must take its share of responsibility.

Terrorism appeals to the media spectacle, to visual ostentatiousness. Therefore we condemn 9/11 as a universal tragedy. Terror loves the camera. Firm evidence: the videos of suicide bombers versus the hand-written suicide note. Two fundamentally different modes of being. Two incompatible ideologies. Suicide bombers display an Extrovert-Supremacist bravado.

Examine the very real problem in today's world of Islamic Extrovert-Supremacism: The American Al–Shabaab fighter Omar Hammami with his spoken word rap and Twitter addiction. The Daesh/ISIS states taking it to the next level with slickly-produced Hollywoodesque productions. Ask yourself: would ISIS ever make a zine with scissors, staples and felt–tips? Herein lies the essence of the problem. The composer Stockhausen disappointed us in comparing 9/11 to a work of art. True composition is internal life.

Insurgent groups that refuse to engage in dialogue are not to be considered terrorist groups. It is resistance in a global system predicated on the 'spokesperson' as the exclusive representative of global democracy.

THE EXTROVERT STATE IS A TERRORIST STATE

The Extrovert World Order at present is the greatest purveyor of terrorism in the world.

States are the prime mover of Extrovert-Supremacist terrorism. The bombing of the Ottoman library in Sarajevo by the Serbian army during the war in the former Yugoslavia was an example of this. So was the looting of the Museum in Iraq during its 'liberation' administered by the American invader. Extrovert-Supremacist ideas are mirrored in media-show formats: the Oprah Winfrey talk show format, the Pop Idol Karaoke format and the Lad Mag are all genres that paved the way towards Extrovert-Supremacist Imperialist domination.

After acts of supreme Extrovert terrorism such as the bombing of Afghanistan in 2001, media displays of Extrovert-Supremacism were used as propaganda to market 'victory'. Look at, for example, the Afghan version of Pop Idol, Afghan Star, or the fashion show catwalk paraded on CNN as an example of the 'liberation' of 'oppressed' subjects.

Shy Radicals reject the recent attempt by the Extrovert World Order (under the influence of the McCarthyite think-tank the Vegas Foundation, embedded in the Establishment) to place it on a list of proscribed terrorist organisations. This has harmed charitable donations to our organisation. We believe The Charity Commission should not be influenced by the Vegas Foundation. This case is currently subject to judicial review. Prisoners claiming association with the movement have had our literature and political material confiscated. In a bid to secure respectibility, Basque's ETA and Ireland's Sinn Féin have publicly distanced themselves from the Shy Radicals Celtic delegation.

We do not accept the terms of civic engagement of Extrovert-Supremacist states. Shy Radicals is a national liberation and resistance organisation, and, when pushed, adopts the strategy of guerrilla operations, sabotage and infiltration. We engage in underground autonomous activities. Shy Radicals harnesses the power of quiet. Audre Lorde said 'silence will not protect you.' And she was wrong.

Our guerrilla resistance and defence strategy are guided by the philosophy of Abu adh-Dhiyal who teaches us:

> 'Learn to be quiet just as you learn to talk, because if talking guides you, being quiet protects you. By being quiet, you attain two characteristics: you are able to take knowledge from those more knowledgeable than you, and you are able to repel the ignorance of those more ignorant than you.'

FIVE

INTERVIEW WITH
SHY RADICALS
POLITICAL PRISONER
AMY LITTLEWOOD

INTERVIEW WITH SHY RADICALS
POLITICAL PRISONER AMY LITTLEWOOD

Amy Littlewood (b. 1968) is the longest detained-without-trial Shy Radicals political prisoner. Held in twenty-three-hour 'company confinement' for thirteen consecutive years, she is subjected to a litany of in-cell video trivialities, experimental small-talk interrogation methods, and suffocated with a sensory overstimulation of chatter noise, with a combined stink of vomit, cheap alcohol and street urine prior to interrogation. Concerns have been raised about the conditions of her pre-trial detention but she is still not officially recognised as a political prisoner, a prisoner of war or a prisoner of conscience by established Western human rights NGOs. Constitutional lawyers and civil liberties campaigners have litigated for better prison conditions, with their fight resulting in Amy's very first public interview in over a decade.

Amy is an Australian national but refuses to fully accept her citizenship status, declaring herself to be a citizen of 'the Aspergistan homeland state'. She was first arrested in 2012 at a United Nations summit for destroying the drafts declaring 2015 the UNESCO year of the Introvert where the cultural contribution of Autistic Spectrum disorders was recognised. Her role in instigating a boycott of the International Introvert Festival of Celebrating Neurodiversity was cited as further grounds for Amy's arrest. She has also received an extradition request from Seoul, South Korea, due to her attempts during 2012 to stop the viral spread of Gangnam-style videos across global social media networks.

She was interviewed in the presence of her radical human rights lawyer Lynne Peirce. The journalist conducting the interview has chosen to remain anonymous but works for an internet and technology magazine. This is the first time the interview has been published in English.

At the time of the interview, Ms Littlewood was in a grey prison uniform, having gained the constitutional right to no longer wear a bright orange jumpsuit (and prior to that a bright yellow jumpsuit) through a recent landmark legal victory at the Supreme Court, which recognised that her 'ethnic rights' as an Introvert had been violated by the imposition of loud colours.

Parts of the interview remain censored for legal reasons.

Q. MS LITTLEWOOD, HOW ARE YOU HOLDING TOGETHER AND SURVIVING?

My lawyer has gradually won me better conditions, setting some legal precedents for all of us surviving the struggle. We Introvert people know how to withdraw into our caves even under the most suffocating and intense forms of 'company confinement'. The prison-like real world of the Extrovert World Order – the world of compulsory parties and commercial suffocation – prepared me for this hell.

I have been denied the right to the university programme. The authorities force me into the company of the most talkative and outgoing prisoners. They invented these torture methods for us, the Shy Underground political prisoners.

I have received thousands of letters of solidarity from around the world. At times, I have had my correspondence withheld from me and have been chained and locked in the card-playing room or the recreation room which resembles a football pitch. Worst of all, they coerce me into looking like I am enjoying myself. The flashing lights, vomit and alcohol-breath I have been subject to are all part of a psychological strategy designed by the state services to resemble the smell of the decadent Extrovert Supremacist Western republics, found for example wafting through the London Underground train carriages and through high streets on Friday and Saturday nights.

They will never understand our feelings of humiliation, rejection and alienation. They talk so much about integration and assimilation, and yet they will not admit that their very insistence on us fitting in is responsible for our radicalisation; it is nothing less than a declaration of war on our peoples.

What gives me strength? The revitalisation of the art of letter-writing amongst our global people is something. In the age of the flash mob and the socialite the renewal of interest in the art of letter-writing is a source of strength and hope. It is a crucial part of the struggle, taken up as an everyday tactic of resistance to the colonisation of time and space by Extrovert-Supremacy.

Q: WHAT HAS THIS EXPERIENCE OF BEING SENT TO PRISON TAUGHT YOU?

Extrovert-Supremacy courses through the criminal justice system and through criminology. You notice this in the media portrayal of convicted criminals: whether it's a murderer, a rapist, or, increasingly, a 'terrorist' or 'domestic extremist', the guilty party is always a 'loner'. And the innocent victim is always 'gregarious', 'popular', a party-lover ready to appear in one of a few stock media narratives. Take the reporting of a recent murder of nine people by white extremist Chris Harper-Mercer at an Oregon USA college campus: in the Associated Press Harper-Mercer was described as 'withdrawn'; a 'quiet loner' who 'seemed really unfriendly' and would 'sit by himself in the dark in the balcony with this little light'. Or, in 1999, the Columbine High School massacre was blamed on goth subculture. The perpetuation of these narratives by the Extrovert media class effectively demarcates the dangerous zone of the Shy 'weirdo'. No one should want to be friends with anyone inhabiting this zone: its people are stigmatised and cannot be accepted as children, students, or members of the community.

In the reporting of murder and acts of terrorism, journalistic standards are swept aside to make room for hearsay. What is driving this? A bid to foster fear and distrust; to stigmatise and criminalise our peoples' histories, identities, roots and ways of being. The mental health system is no better, also used as an instrument of oppression. My experience is that my life – led according to my Introvert ways – has always been associated with mental ill health. Why is it that participation in Trendy Club is propagated as the embodiment of 'health'? Empirical data collected by our research wing shows that party girl behaviours result in more ill health and psychological vulnerability. Social anxiety disorder is 'cured' by a pseudo-chemical fix. But what would it mean to be cured? The medics pathologise our peoples but we should instead, as the Socialist Patients' Collective advised, use illness as our weapon.

Q: TELL ME HOW YOU WENT FROM BEING AN AUSTRALIAN STUDENT ACTIVIST TO, AS SOME WOULD SAY, THE CATALYST OF THE SHY RADICALS MOVEMENT?

For a start, I would like to say I do not recognise Australia, nor do I recognise myself as an 'Aussie'. I would never be seen drinking Fosters at a 'barbie'. Extrovert 'democracy', the world of PR projectionism and salesmanship may be spreading like a virus but we need to cure the disease. The cure is the state of Aspergistan, and the refusal of its people to be co-opted into the system...

It was the system that started it all, in fact, when they closed my local library and took away my favourite park bench. I was left without a place to sit and watch the ducks, sometimes feeding them homemade bread. All the quiet havens were replaced by noisy shopping centres, nightclubs and Trendy bars. It was too much. But it was also my awakening.

I had read about many UK-wide campaigns against the 'regeneration' of local communities; at first, Shy Radicals formed an alliance with them. This was initially attended by the Elderly Peoples Association (not all of whom were of an Introvert intersectional political persuasion) and reported only in local news media. But the effects of the Extrovert-Supremacist system began to be felt nationally: forests, cathedrals and yet more local libraries disappeared. The system's 'regeneration schemes' transformed the high streets into channels for Extrovert-Supremacist vomit and urine, which came flowing out of endless Extrovert-Supremacist-exclusive venues. The entire public sphere evolved to meet Extrovert-Supremacist demands. Churches turned into nightclubs: Mass was just one such place in London, formerly St. Mathew's Church located in the Peace Gardens of Brixton Hill. The conversion of the crypt into a venue accommodating up to 1,500 clubbers at once was somehow declared to be in the public interest. I mourn for this, not because I have any interest in the institutional power of Christianity but because I understand what is really being lost. The war on piety is not about institutional religion as such; rather it is about the cleansing of my people and about the destruction of our way of life. During my early days at the Introverts Rights Association, I fought for the transformation of public space to be recognised as a form of 'discrimination'. Only the most half-hearted kind of legislation was introduced. The 'multi-cultural' forum refused to help us – placing Extrovert-Supremacists in the LGBT and Black communities with whom we were aligned. The forum just didn't get where we were coming from – they would say: well, some of my best friends are Shy people. But they were missing the point, blinded by their Extrovert-liberalism. We need to stick it to the Man.

Q: NOT ALL SHY PEOPLE BELIEVE IN THE SYSTEM OF SHYRIA LAW.

BUT YOU HAVE SAID THAT IT IS MANDATORY FOR ALL SHY PEOPLE TO SUPPORT THIS?

WHY IS THIS SO?

When I was free, I came to realise that there was just nowhere for Shy people to go on a Friday night. I walked and walked around the Brixton area looking for just a quiet, low-lit place to sit and have a meaningful face-to-face conversation with my friend. Just one place. But everywhere we went, all around the high streets and the backstreets and the markets, every place was rammed, bustling, pumping out incessant noise. This was supposed to be a sign of a 'lively' and 'successful' area. But before we even walked through the door of one bar after another… surely you can imagine the unhomeliness of them all.

So I began to wonder whether quiet places could be legally protected, whether their preservation could be made statutory. Could legal rights be introduced to acknowledge our way of being? In the interests of Shy relations, could space in the public sphere be reserved in alignment with our needs? Could that be conceivable? Could it be a realistic demand?

Such hopes begin to fade when you realise that the entire legislative body is made up of people of a certain personality. They are supposed to represent you but there are no shy people among them. And our people don't stand a chance of entering their ranks: they don't have the 'personality' to run for election, leaving the people with 'personality' to speak on our behalf. As if they can! They only speak to their own class… You begin to ask yourself: what changes would be necessary here?

I remember when the question entered my head. A police siren had just zoomed passed us in the streets and we realised how the presence of the state makes itself felt through repetitive, piercing noise and flashing light. The state apparatus itself is imitative of extroversion. In fact it reinforces the social and political order, supplementing noise with more noise. How can you expect the state to protect you?

Q: THE SHY RADICAL MOVEMENT WAS INITIALLY CALLED THE SHY PEOPLE'S PANTHER PARTY.

WHY THE CHANGE?

I initially took inspiration from the Black Panthers. I see Shy Radicals as the Black Panthers of the Introvert class.

We initially changed our cell name to the Shy Underground, and then this became the name of our Autistic Spectrums operations wing, after a note was passed around in the prison library. We remembered the lessons from history: even the Black Panthers degenerated into an Extrovert-Supremacist movement. 'Angelina Davis' was the term I coined for this phenomenon, whereby celebrity overtakes commitment and substance. The former freedom fighters who often put themselves in the firing line, some crippled by their prison experiences, now indluge themselves with extortionate speakers' fees. Like supermodels, they will not get out of bed for less than thousands of dollars. Check the content of their speech, now diluted to the platitudes of Liberal NGOs: what is the difference between what they're saying and other forms of Hollywood celebrity endorsement?

We reject the phenomenon of 'Shysters' too, hanging out at cafes and choosing so-called 'lifestyle shyness' – just like an American college kid wearing a Che Guevara T-shirt. Meaningless... we see this too in the adoption of the Black Power afro by Trendy Club. All these so-called arts from below: slam poetry, graffiti art, or even the macho bravado of gangsta rap? They steal our language, telling people about all the things they 'dig' – using this word as a 'cool' form of street slang. But we Shy Radicals really *dig*: we investigate, plunging into the depths and diving for treasure – denying shallowness and superficiality is the basis of our politics. The Black Liberation narrative has culminated in Extrovert-Supremacist icons like Beyoncé and Afro-Zionism, basketball stars and Black Capitalism. I reject it all. It offends me as a woman. What is really at play is not any single issue of race, class or gender but Extrovert-Supremacist chauvinism as a whole; the Extrovert class trying to sell a liberation narrative or story of empowerment to the Shy and still oppressed.

Q: WHAT IS MEANT BY TRENDY CLUB? IT IS A TERM THAT APPEARS MOST FREQUENTLY IN YOUR PRISON WRITINGS.

I said previously that Trendy Club is not just a building that functions as a discotheque but something insidious, something that shapes the world order. Trendy Club is not just something to do on a weekend as a distracting pastime: it is an ideology and monoculture.

It permeates the whole of society, its images, behaviour, values and subjectivity, its perceptions. Everywhere – look around you in the streets at how people dress, how they govern their behaviour, how they love or hate themselves. Trendy Club is inescapable now... the banality of its evil. Try going out to buy a pair of shoes from the high street; the chances are that an Extrovert feel-good tune will be blasting through the speakers, specially selected by the 'outgoing personality' of the person fitting the shoes. The shoes themselves will have been marketed in full-on Extrovert format, appearing on celebrity-emblazoned billboards. And the celebrities themselves will have acquired their power through their 100-per-cent commitment to the Extrovert Power structure. Try simply buying a coffee or a sandwich and the story will be the same.

Time itself is defined, governed and colonised by the Friday. Extrovert-Supremacists maintain the alienating routine of the working week. They live for their Friday night release, their complicity justifying the sheep-like zombie death they endure every other weekday. Friday night is to be spent in the manner dictated by Trendy Club, which has colonised the future too, projecting a teleological picture of human history. For imperialists, Trendy Club is the image of the finally liberated man: the aspirational site of liberated humanity.

Afghanistan was invaded so that a Trendy Club system could be established there. It makes us feel like second-class citizens and it is an apartheid system for our youth – those who go to Trendy Club will be elevated. Sadly, those who are left behind will carry an inferiority complex with them throughout their high school and college days. They will be marooned and rejected because Trendy Club cultivates man's very worst traits: shallowness, vanity, arrogance, sexual chauvinism, ostentatiousness. Trendy Club's locales are factories of triviality, and include some of the rowdiest pubs, where a sports result or celebrity gossip is discussed with greater urgency than ongoing genocide and war.

Whilst the Extrovert-class calls *us* boring and dull, you have to wonder at the dullness of the Extrovert class itself. If they enjoy themselves so much, why is it that they have to take so many photographs of themselves, submitting them to Instagram and Facebook as 'proof'? In the study of such acts, we have discovered a type of Extrovert blandness. Imagine the blurring and blending together of all the iPhone photos of Extrovert-Supremacists posing in horrible Trendy Club bars across the world. Imagine them all beginning to look exactly the same as one another... But wait a minute, that's how it already is [laughs]. Ask yourself: why does Paris Hilton exist? Purely and solely for Trendy Club.

Q: THE CHAIR OF THE INTROVERTS RIGHTS ASSOCIATION ED NAWAZ HAS REQUESTED TO VISIT YOU IN PRISON. BUT YOU HAVE DECLINED.

WHY IS THIS?

The Introverts Rights Association was absorbed by state-funded government programmes a long time ago, and now has several Extroverts – including an auctioneer, a club DJ and a fashion model – on its board of trustees and amongst its staff. Absolute betrayal... They even accepted PREVENT funding to continue their work. We are not playing that game. We set our own rules. We establish our own ways of defining ourselves. We live rich introspective lives, and refuse to be governed according to the same market forces that let American college movies proliferate. Let alone 'reclaim' them as some House Introverts do.

We refuse to recognise all Extrovert-Supremacist parliaments and law systems. We wish to be governed by our own system - the legislation of Shyria law – the law drafted by Shy, Introvert and Autistic spectrum peoples' political representatives only. Shy-autonomy: the right to self-determination. No more exploitation by the Extrovert class.

The Introvert Rights Association chair and I were comrades from our college days. I no longer recognise him. There will be no real Introvert rights until the entire Trendy Club system is abolished and the last outgoing person is hung by the wires of their sound systems. I admit, we co-edited the party newspaper, *The Hedgehog Fire*, and even authored some academic papers together. It is said that he received funding for a new think tank – the so-called Vegas Foundation – by declaring himself an ex-Shy Radical, and claiming that 'our' goal had simply been integration and the maintenance of a 'negative peace'. He encourages us to tolerate the unjust order, to live on our knees, to iron out all insurgence into compliance. He has since been accepted onto state-funded public programmes around University campuses: a form of neo-McCarthyism that sees him preying on quiet students. The subversives and deviants who 'spend too much time alone in their bedrooms' were reported to the authorities. The snitch, the traitor! Ed even supported turning the library archives of the University of Manchester into a student karaoke bar.

I still support the inclusion of Introvert History Month in the local council, prison service and secondary school calendar, while Ed sees his crowning achievement as establishing the first Introvert Studies programme at University of California, Berkeley in the postcolonial Studies department. I agree that our heritage, the proto-Shy Radicals, our icons of resistance: Rosa Parks, Blaise Pascal, Emily Dickinson, Wednesday Addams, and Lisa Simpson must be reclaimed in our canon. But for a real Shy Radical, every day is Introvert History Month.

Q: WHY DOES THE SHY RADICALS PARTY STILL BOYCOTT THE FESTIVAL OF NEURO-DIVERSITY?

Divide and rule is their game. First, the authorities attempted to divide us into various pathologies: Asperger's syndrome, social anxiety disorder, depression. But we are all one. We suffer as one. We fight as one. And then it was 'extremist' introverts and 'moderate' introverts. They want to depoliticise Shyness as a purely 'cultural phenomenon' or a medical pathology. Worse than that, they want to present us as the United Colours of Benetton of personality types. They want Little Miss Quiet here, and Cute Little Fragile boy there, Mr. Clumsy here and Little Johnny Goofy there. They want us to accept the taxonomies of their diagnostic manuals like an aviary of exotic birds. But shyness is a political position.

When the Introverts Rights Association settled for a minimal state-funded programme of Celebrating Neurodiversity, and no more – he compromised himself and the Shy Radical community. It was like Yasser Arafat signing the Oslo Accords; or Martin McGuinness shaking hands with the Queen.

We also note the festival of Neurodiversity's invitation of the traitor Susan Cain. Author of the book *Quiet: The Power of Introverts in a World That Can't Stop Talking* (2012), Cain is a sell-out and darling of the Extrovert circuit. She is seen as representing us all, but all she did was note down some of the structural features of the Extrovert system, the way that Extrovert-Supremacism plays out, for example, in employment and marketing. She loves to say that Shy people are not Introverts, and that Introverts are not Shy. She is a collaborator in the game of divide and rule. We have suffered in the same way. We are a united front. I admit that when I first watched her TED talks, I had a teenage crush. I was in love with her... until she said 'my husband is an Extrovert'. It ripped me apart. She was literally sleeping with the enemy. Her book is just stats that fuel the corporate management system that keeps us out of work: pseudoscience and bad research. Susan Cain is a corporate lawyer and mere hobbyist who has left her people behind. What we need is a proper scientific Shy Radicalism and a vanguard resistance movement, true to its roots. She plays the token Introvert.

Boycott in itself is one of the key Shy Radical tactics: withdrawal is the most powerful weapon. I proposed a motion at the Introfada summit that all Susan Cain's events should be boycotted.

Oh dear God, these days there is a whole new industry built around psychology and self-help books spurred by Susan Cain's TED talk popularity! Sometimes the odd well-meaning Extrovert Liberal will send these kinds of publication to me in prison... I confess I cringe or roll my eyes... Titles include

How to Survive in an Extrovert World, and worse still, there is a business management book called *The Introvert Advantage: How Introverts can Thrive in an Extrovert World*. Authors are often 'qualified' in the academic field of psychology, or they hold an MBA. There is another trend, a subgenre of pop-Buddhism that stresses the health benefits of mindfulness in our world of noise.

Why do they assume in the first instance that the world belongs to Extroverts?

Do they think that the world should be Extrovert?

Do they believe that us Introverts just want to get along, content with a place that has been set as low as that of peasants in a medieval painting?

And if they truly believe that the world cannot be changed will this perception exist until the end of time?

Q: FOLLOWING ON FROM THAT POINT, IS SHY RADICALS TO BE UNDERSTOOD AS AN ANTI-CAPITALIST MOVEMENT?

We feel betrayed by the anti-capitalist and anti-globalisation movement for its failure to recognise the forces of imperialism are driven by monopoly extroversion. Our North Japan and North Korea delegations have much more to say on this. Cuba meanwhile is complicit in Extrovert promotion – with its revolution and party tourist trap. Irish Leftist Republicanism has degenerated into green-tinted plastic pub singalongs. Emma Goldman's 'If I can't dance, I don't want to be part of your revolution' demands a total subversion, too: *if* you dance, we do not want to be part of yours.

You also have to question why the opposite of the World Economic Forum is called the World *Social* Forum. As if socialising were inherently emancipatory? If that's the case then every

Kardashian and every two-bit socialite, gossip-rag airhead is part of the 'emancipation' narrative. Worse, though, is 'Reclaim the Streets' - samba bands, and the hollow hedonism of political rave party 'culture'.

Aside from this collaborationist tendency, we note that when Leninist parties spoke of 'disciplined' criticism in their manifestos they did so in a bid to temper the flux of voices. Party discipline was latent Shy Radicalism.

Q: THE INDICTMENT THAT YOU ARE CURRENTLY CONTESTING CLAIMS THAT SHY RADICALS IS RECEIVING FUNDING FROM NORTH KOREA.

CAN YOU COMMENT ON THIS?

As the case is going to trial, I can't comment on any details of this confidential matter which is currently under discussion with my lawyer.

And I will say that the Korean War is one of the most misunderstood of all twentieth century conflicts. It is neither a Cold War hangover nor a clash of communist and capitalist ideology. The hermit kingdom has in the past offered me shelter, refuge and diplomatic immunity.

There are two Koreas at war: Korea with its ornate Buddhist monasteries and Zen palaces, stones and cool running streams, and Korea with its growing world of K-pop and plastic malls. South Korea is a victim of Trendy Club ideology and is nothing less than a devil's playground. Ever since its integration into global capitalism there has been neon, neon everywhere: in the hyper-karaoke bars with their flashing lights, in holographic advertising and in shopping malls kept open 24/7. We can see the roots of the conflict if we pay close attention to South Korean psychological warfare, which is encapsulated in the weapon of mass distraction of the 'Gangnam Style' global conspiracy. When the music video for Psy's 'Gangnam Style' hit over one billion views on YouTube in 2012 we saw proof of the pervasiveness of Extrovert-Supremacism. In the world of globalised media, it might be compared to a landmark such as Hitler's invasion of Poland. Simply put, the real reason for the continuation of decades of hostilities and the cycles of mutual nuclear weapon antagonism with North Korea is just because, as a nation, it is a bit shy.

WHY DOES THE SHY RADICAL MOVEMENT REFUSE TO RECOGNISE ISRAEL?

One army – the resistance forces of the Palestinian people – conducts combat via underground tunnels. The Israeli Defence Force carries out its operations via sonic booms, flying planes with ear-shattering clamour and bombs, imposing noise as a weapon of war. It should be clear from that alone, which party should be seen as legitimate and compatible with the Shy Radical vision of the future.

Tel Aviv is the nightclub capital of Israel and spreads Extrovert-Supremacism in the West Asian region. Israel is an apartheid state and yet there was a media stunt showing Palestinians dancing alongside members of the Israeli Defence Force in a version of 'Gangnam Style'. Is this the final destination of the Nakbah? What thousands went on hunger strike to achieve? This is what they call 'peace-building.' We refuse to recognise Israel's right to exist. I don't need to say anymore.

Q: IN ACADEMIC WORK PRODUCED BY THE MOVEMENT, THERE IS TALK THAT SHY PEOPLE NEED TO INVENT A NEW LANGUAGE.

CAN YOU COMMENT ON THIS?

The movement began life as a school of literary theory. It brought attention to how the structure of language itself is predicated upon Extrovert-Supremacy. A question commonly posed by the global Left is: 'Why don't you call yourself a *bold* radical?' As if Shyness operated in binary opposition to 'bold', with shyness as the absent or deficient term. Shyness for Shy Radicals is the like word 'Black' for adherent of Black Power. Similarly, when the prison authorities throw around that I am 'reserved', it bears no resemblance to the reality of our world. The authorities make deviants of us. There is nothing reserved or held back or behind-the-barrier. We are at peace with ourselves. It's just that our reality is made to seem bleak by the Extrovert-Supremacists' compulsion to talk without stopping; their mouths like toilets over-spilling into the world.

In their letters, my supporters tell me that there is a place in London called 'Speakers' Corner' – an area of a public park where Extroverts stand. But why do the people not notice the corner instead of the speaker? We speak from the corner.

Q: OUR PRISON VISIT TIME IS RUNNING OUT.

ANY FINAL COMMENTS?

Extrovert-Supremacists confuse their lifestyle with life itself; and our privileging of inner contemplation, slowness and depth of reflection with death. Our condition of subjugation has seen us suffering thousands of bullying, derogatory words and thousands of American college movies, especially during the Reagan and Thatcher years. We teach life; they teach zombification, numbness, shallowness, posing, hollowness. The world of Trendy Club is an oppressive world of posers, materialism, compulsive consumption, lovelessness, networked vanity. Theirs is a world of infinite distraction. Another world is possible...

Free all Shy Radical political prisoners...

[AMY LITTLEWOOD IS ESCORTED AWAY BY PRISON GUARDS.]

End of interview.

SIX

BUILDING THE SHY RADICAL STUDENT MOVEMENT

A quiet kid was bullied at school for the mere fact of being quiet. There was no -ism or historical legacy he could turn to or seek hope within. There was no subgroup of hate crime legislation he could turn to. There was no lobby group campaigning for the rights, suitable living and labour conditions of quiet people. Unlike other forms of hate crime, there are no statistics accounting for the painful experiences that quiet people have been through. Yet, I feel, the problem is privately acknowledged on a massive scale.

– Transcription from the first Shy Radical student movement meeting

Reports from the Introvert Rights Association Domestic Crisis Centre illustrate that many Shy people do not survive their early experiences of school or are left scarred and traumatised. This situation is exacerbated by the increasing commodification of what Extrovert-Supremacists identify as 'Youth Culture'. University and college life are promoted as centres of 'Youth Culture' and are dominated by Extrovert-Supremacist elites. Introvert hate crime is rife within secondary school and college, decreasing somewhat at higher levels of university study. Teachers can be complicit in the ill-treatment of Shy people, noting in Shy persons' school reports that their alternative modes of communication are 'cause for concern'.

Shy Radicals recognise the necessity of building a Shy Radical Student Movement. The failure of 'diversity' initiatives offered the labels of intersectionality: Women's officer, Black officer and LGBT officers at National Union of Students level are self-evident. In all cases, they misrepresent us, as they are dominated in all cases by their leadership structure and are elected in such ways that mean the odds are stacked against Shy candidates. Diversity initiatives also foster forms of celebration and participation that alienate Shy Radicals, who additionally reject the offer of the National Student Union president that Shyness be recognised as a disability.

The student union is an obstacle in our path to liberation.

A breakaway Aspergistan Student Organisation (ASO) was attempted, promoting the history and cultures of introvert life. This also attracted excessive criticism and concerted hostility, with accusation of 'atomisation' and 'sectarianism' between other radical political student societies. The word 'Aspergistan' has sometimes been anonymously defaced and is subject of abusive toilet graffiti on campus. Many of the National Union of Students leadership have mistaken Aspergistan as a Muslim organisation (as many national representative bodies such as the Pakistan, Palestine and Afghanistan societies exist). Much to our bemusement, our student representatives found themselves programmed to speak during Islamophobia Awareness Month. We are still investigating whether this was an accidental or deliberate error on behalf of the student administration.

The list of universities that have passed a Shy Radicals student union motion are placed on the central website. Whilst passing a motion is welcome, the objective at stake is a radical reconstitution of the student body to halt the spread of Extrovert internal colonisation of student campuses, accommodation halls and university life.

Our objective is to create a sense of empowerment amongst the non-Extrovert students. Our object is to let our grievances be known and to dictate the terms of engagement.

The leadership of neuro-typical student movements at present remains unsympathetic to all Shy Radical demands, which were rejected wholesale at the National Union of Students AGM.

WE DEMAND... CURRICULUM REFORM

Shyness features excessively in degree programmes such as psychology with an emphasis on Shyness as a problem to be overcome via assertiveness skills and cognitive retraining. It sums up our place in this society. This needs immediate wholesale reform.

We need to put Shyness at the heart of undergraduate, post-graduate and postdoctoral programmes such as sociology, politics, history, geography, philosophy and international relations. Arenas such as linguistics and language need to recognise us. And finally, we need to find a way of being acknowledged into histories of art, science, literatures and the history of thought.

OVERTURN… WAR WITHIN: INTROVERTS AGAINST CUTS

1   Staff/student ratios have progressively worsened. Introvert students are thus forced into large-scale, party-like, company-suffocating classrooms where their voices are often drowned out by loudmouthed Extrovert-Supremacists. This is an ideological attack on the preference for small company by Introvert peoples in an attempt to disempower us. This is an enormous loss to Introvert participation in the classroom and lecture theatre. Equality to quiet students is denied.

2   Cuts to the budgets of university libraries as well as limiting their hours of access, just as at national grassroots level, can be seen part of the concerted war against our peoples. Shy Radicals aspire to twenty-four-hour library access as well as total freedom to organise meetings for the Aspergistan international movement. The Dewey Decimal system of classification is also being investigated by the Shy Radical research wing as to whether or not it is a structurally Extrovert-System: this may result in an alternative taxonomy being drafted. The Harvard referencing system has also been subject to the same scrutiny.

3   A lectern is not a podium. These constitute two different modes of engagement. Shy Radicals wholeheartedly reject that the podium speaker constitutes a figure of mass representation. Shy Radicals will not tolerate the abuse of the university lectern as a podium.

BUILDING THE SHY RADICAL STUDENT MOVEMENT

AUTODIDACTICISM

Shy Radicals encourage maximum participation in higher levels of the institutionalisation of learning and its dissemination into non-institutionalised public life. There remains an internal debate within the party about the value of autodidacticism and non-institutionalised learning. There exists a lingering feeling of betrayal about new university disciplines such as cultural studies which was felt to legitimise Extrovert-Supremacist pratices and ascribe 'non-hierarchical' emancipatory politics to its cultural manifestations.

STOP… CAMPUS MCCARTHYISM: STUDENTS NOT SUSPECTS

Solidarity with Shy Radicals political prisoners has also been targeted and blacklisted by watchdogs and the think-tank the Vegas Foundation. There are also internal fears that the organisation will decay into a conformist organisation in a bid merely to survive. Students who decide to stay in their rooms have been treated suspiciously by the authorities as potential subversives and deviants.

A Shy Radical student newspaper entitled *The Room* is to be published and distributed soon.

ACKNOWLEDGE… THE SCHIZOPHRENIA OF STUDENT LIFE

Entry into student life at once features a contradiction for Shy, Introvert and Autistic Spectrum peoples: a bipolar experience. At one end, the peak of introspection and depths of study; at the other, a potentially painful experience at the peak of vulnerbility: likely to be a victim of Extrovert harassment, company suffocation, compulsory alcohol intake, public humiliation, initiation into Trendy Club and its ensuing totally decadent ideology. The security and dignity of the Shy peoples are not protected. Rather, they are put, intentionally, at risk, under the guise of 'team participation' and 'leisure facilities'.

Peer pressure to imitate and emulate the Extrovert-hedonist lifestyle should be seen in the light of cultural self-hatred. Introvert students also find themselves blamed for the alcohol-fuelled public disorder caused by Extrovert students' lifestyle choices in city centres, whilst remaining entirely innocent.

Shy Radicals students often have high expectations of university, having earlier been subject to forms of compulsory groupthink, a compulsory participative form in primary and secondary schools.

I am suffocating, drowning.
Oh the college.
SOS...
Everyone around me is too outgoing to notice...
Give me a window of hope...
there is nothing to turn to.
No exit.
Descend down Shy Peoples' Student Movement
– protect me...

– Excerpt from the suicide note of a young Shy Radicals martyr from the Crisis Voices archives, who gassed himself to death in his student hall kitchen.

The most potent weapon of the oppressor is the mind of
the oppressed.

– Steve Biko, Anti-Apartheid student leader

Piecemeal adjustment of the institution of education will not do. Rather, these problems must be recognised as wider structural concerns of the Extrovert-Supremacist society. The monopoly of the Extrovert-Supremacist movie industry has been complicit in the rise of stigmatisation and Introvert hate crime amongst young people. Children's television, again led by the penetration of profit, has also had a part to play in bullying and stigmatisation.

REALISE... THE BETRAYAL OF POST-STUDENT LIFE: ADMIN AND THE DESTRUCTION OF INTROVERT LIFE

Trauma is also experienced as a result of the gulf between the stimulating richness of Introvert life experience at university level followed by the internal dullness of postgraduate employment, subservient to Extrovert industry in work environments not adapted to Introvert needs. Introverts often experience feelings of rejection, alienation and worthlessness once put on the job market, and are generally devalued. Faring barely better are those with successive unpaid internships within the cultural industries, increasing subservience to Extrovert-Supremacy under the false guise of 'accessibility'.

SHY CANON

Icons of attainment, aspiration and 'success' that have been provided by the Extrovert establishment such as Bill Gates (of Microsoft) and Steve Jobs (of Apple's consumer base boom) are wholeheartedly rejected by the Shy Radical movement for their complicity in the expansion of corporate capitalism – an economy subservient to the needs of the Extrovert. In the case of Bill Gates, his public posturing with models and celebrities for the selfish pursuit of his own profit is to be condemned by our movement. Apple have also been complicit in the shallow 'Shyster' lifestyle and its aesthetics, co-opted by the ideology of Trendy Club. Collaborators and traitors such as Susan Cain have been complicit in compromising our autonomy.

PLAN OF ACTION

1   Shy Radicals resolves to seek total autonomy in defining our own heroes and icons, and reject all attempts to patronise us by the Extrovert class. Moreover, promotions of such icons have a double nefarious aim, which is to

suggest that integration with the Extrovert-Supremacism system is possible, which we know to be an illusion and false consciousness.

2 Shy Radicals resolves to distribute posters and promotional material relating to Introvert History Month to be displayed in student common rooms.

3 School inspector criteria to be re-evaluated. Reports on the performance and conditions of existing public inspection bodies such as OFSTED to be considered void. A central factor of empirical humiliation must be factored in. Socialist, capitalist and the existing public sector means of assessing education can only seem to be quantified in terms of a development model. That is say that the experience is measured by degrees of literacy in the general citizenry, the provision of technical facilities and increases and decreases in exam results grouped into league tables. The actual nightmarish experience of a high school for our quiet peoples is completely missing. Indeed, it can be completely hidden as long as the technical criteria for assessment are met. We need to configure new taxonomies for assessing the student experience. Bureaucratic bullying policy simply fails to acknowledge the depth of the problem and its systemic nature. This is a task for the future.

4 Abolish the graduation ceremony. The ritual of graduation remains a hangover from a time when the extrovert-class sought to flatten and homogenise the introvert experience. The culmination of in-depth research and investigation cannot be represented by throwing a hat into the air. This is an unhealthy, ingrained extrovert supremacist habit across the board. Serious, fulfilling efforts are treated as the air within a flimsy decorative balloon that must, upon completion, be burst with a pin and disposed of

amidst cheers and laughter. This coerced habit that devalues hours, years and even decades of valuable effort in one fell swoop, must be put to rest for the benefit of what is becoming an increasingly dumbed-down society. People are detached from their roots due to lack of knowledge of what came before. In terms of the graduation ceremony, this problem may be tied into the prior point about the lectern being abused as a public podium. The ritual and closing speeches of each and every one of these ceremonies across universities large and small are synthesised, devaluing individual students and the efforts put in by them. The practice itself, where the Dean of Students or some other, similar senior figure is believed to speak on behalf of all students, belongs to a different time and era, and is utterly unbeneficial. Similar forms of pomp and ceremony exist within the parliamentary chambers and law courts of extrovert-supremacist states where the ritual of powers are maintained through wigs and robes.

The dress of black cloak and hat mocks the rituals of the introvert clergy from twelfth-century Europe (that has since disappeared altogether from mainstream cultural life). The ritual of humiliation should not be recognised as any more legitimate than wearing the 'Red Indian' costume at fancy-dress parties, which is now acknowledged as mocking the genocide of First Nations peoples.

The constitutional fairness of the ceremony is currently being challenged by our movement lawyers. Our student society is also providing support to students who feel under family pressure but choose to opt out of the photograph. The cloak, gown and studio photograph remain archaic and can not be conceived as welcome in an age when introversion must be accepted on equal terms.

PENDING LEGAL CASES

Movement lawyers seek to challenge the imposition of Extrovert social formations on our people within the institution of the university. They currently have the following pending lawsuits:

Jock v. Eliot – a case involving repeated harassment of those who want to stay in their rooms during evening hours, occurring in a student hall of residence.

Sunny University Committee v. Curtis – a case that seeks to limit the use of sitting in a circle – a bid to imitate group therapy – as adopted in secondary school PSHE lessons (offering education on sex and drugs, etc.) as humiliating and inappropriate for the needs of Shy students.

Everyman Emotion Support Department v. Amos – a case concerning a counselling department blaming a client's ill health and chronic depression on lack of integration within the common room and 'nightlife' leisure facilities. A clear case of victim-blaming.

Whilst we wish our movement lawyers every success for standing up for the vulnerable elements of our people, we are fully aware that a loss in the courtroom is not the final word within a legislative system that is structurally against us. Let us be we under no illusion: true justice can not be served as long as extrovert-supremacy governance continues.

CURATING SHY PEOPLE:
SHY RADICALS FILM SEASON
(AND TRAINING FILMS)

SEVEN

CURATING SHY PEOPLE:
SHY RADICALS FILM SEASON
(AND TRAINING FILMS)

SHY RADICALS FILM SEASON
(AND TRAINING FILMS)

The Shy Radicals Film Season was initiated by the Introvert Rights Association at the BFI Southbank. This was a partnership project, overseen by the Social Democrat mayor at the time of a major summer sports event, to showcase the 'rainbow spectrum of the world's greatest city's young people'. Within the party meeting notes, the anonymous scrawling 'mere crumbs' can be found. The mayor's proposal was patronising, and the BFI was far too high-profile a setting for us Shy people, not to mention the extent to which it made a mockery of our struggle by scheduling Hollywood blockbusters throughout the Shy Season.

The faction that eventually broke away from the Introvert Rights Association to form the Shy Radical movement pushed for all Shy Radical student activists to hold an unofficial film season across university campuses, local trade union branches, churches, mosques, and local libraries. The *hikikomori* delegation volunteered to distribute further films, working from their bedrooms to make them available online to other Shy peoples across East Asia. International participation in the unofficial season came to override the Anglophone bias of the earlier selections by the Introvert Rights Association and the BFI. The Shy Radicals and their international networks also rejected the official summertime programming, deciding that their season should be held in the autumn and winter months.

It was also decided that the unofficial programme would be made freely available to Shy people interested in organising small group screenings of the films. Open access would be granted on the understanding that opening galas and red carpets were strictly prohibited, that Autism-friendly environments would be provided, and that all screenings begin with the Shy Radicals' agitprop introduction: a short film documenting the decadence of the Extrovert-Supremacist lifestyle.

FILM PROGRAMME

Silence (2012)
Director: Pat Collins.
Ireland.
83 minutes.

Eoghan is a sound-recordist who returns from Berlin to Donegal, Ireland, for a job capturing sound in areas free from man-made noise. On his journey through remote Irish terrain, he is drawn into a series of encounters and conversations, which gradually divert his attention towards a more intangible silence, bound up with the sounds of the life he had left behind.

Influenced by folklore and making use of archive footage, *Silence* unfolds with a quiet intensity, where poetic images reveal an absorbing meditation on themes relating to sound and silence, history, memory and exile.

Real Fiction (2000)
Director: Kim Ki-duk.
South Korea.
85 minutes.

Joo Jin-mo is a quiet and repressed artist who tolerates an endless stream of humiliating abuse from customers and street thugs as he sketches portraits in a park. Through an encounter with a dissatisfied customer, Joo finds himself enraged by the reality of his life and becomes hell-bent on tracking down everyone who has ever tormented him. Unfortunately for the individuals who so frivolously wronged this fragile artist, a simple apology will not suffice and bloodlust can only be satisfied with blood. Joo is determined by means of murderous retaliation to reverse the damage done to his soul. He is completely unaware, however, that someone is secretly recording his killing spree, capturing it all with a camcorder.

A Night of Prophecy (2002)
Director: Amar Kanwar.
India.
77 minutes.

The film chronicles nationalist separatist struggles through India from Kashmir to Naga peoples though their poetry and folksongs. The film shows how hushed, reflective quiet can be a positive indication of cultural resistance or of an impending political transformation.

Sunny (2011)
Director: Kang Hyeong-cheol.
South Korea.
124 minutes.

A shy and quiet girl, Na-mi, arrives in a strange new town, where she instantly becomes the target of her new school's bullies. Out-numbered and with nowhere to turn, Na-mi is suddenly saved by a bizarre, misfit group of girls. Though their friendship grows strong, a terrible accident rips them asunder for twenty-five years. As an adult Na-mi regrets the way things turned out and looks to bring the misfit group back together.

Temple Grandin (2010)
Director: Mick Jackson.
USA.
107 mins.

The film focuses on the Autistic icon, writer and scientist Temple Grandin, celebrating her life and contribution to the liberation of Autistic Spectrum peoples.

13 Lakes / Ten Skies (2004)
Director: James Benning.
USA.
135 minutes.

Benning's deceptively simple titles – *13 Lakes* and *Ten Skies* – belie the richly nuanced worlds of light, shadow, stillness, and change in each film's ten-minute shot. Structurally and conceptually minimalist, *13 Lakes* presents thirteen bodies of water from across the United States – each chosen for its unique historical, ecological and geographical characteristics, and each framed to divide the image evenly between water and sky. *Ten Skies* adopts a similar format with the camera turned directly upward to the formation of clouds and aerial life. The precision and rigour of the film's form intensifies the experience of duration, with Benning's long takes embracing both his subject (to which he is acutely attentive) and his audience (to whom he generously offers the time for audio-visual immersion), inviting us to share in his sober contemplation of the ever-subtly shifting mystery of the natural world. On the occasion of the Shy Radicals Film Season, selected works by Stan Brakhage were shown before and after Benning's films. Among them, *Mothlight* (1963) was selected for its demonstration of Brakhage's acute sensitivity to colour and for its experimental means of production – without a camera. Created using clear packing tape, which Brakhage used to collect moths' wings, flower petals, leaves, dust, and other ephemeral natural debris, *Mothlight* is a beautiful and brief meditation on life and death from one of the masters of 'visionary' film. Also selected for the season is Brakhage's 1971 body of silent films known as *The Pittsburgh Trilogy: Eyes* documents Brakhage's ride through Pittburgh in a police car; *Deus Ex* is filmed in a hospital as part of the director's attempt to overcome his fear of the medical institution; *The Act of Seeing with One's Own Eyes* takes the camera into the autopsy room.

TRAINING FILMS:

The following films will be shown as part of a recruitment and training programme for all new Shy Radical members.

Heathers (1988)
Director: Michael Lehmann.
USA.
102 minutes.
Starring: Winona Ryder, Christian Slater, Shannen Doherty.

Original notes, first delivered in a training camp lecture series in an Afghan cave and preserved for the Introvert Archive studies programme: The 1980s American college movie *Heathers* must be understood, first and foremost, as a political film. The film's central protagonists, Veronica (Winona Ryder) and JD (Christian Slater), represent two positions on the Shy political spectrum: Veronica exhibits the reformist tendency and JD the revolutionary. The film documents the consciousness-raising efforts of Veronica, a teenage student fighting for the oppressive conditions and Extrovert-Supremacist class hierarchy of the high school to be recognised and redressed.

The film *Heathers*, initially a commercial flop in the cinema, found new life on the VHS format through private small-scale screenings, and is constantly being revived by individuals streaming the film online. Almost thirty years after its release, the film has achieved a cult following and a place in the Introvert canon. It attempts to subvert the American college movie genre, taking it in a darker direction via the topic of serial teenage suicide.

(It is worth noting that the American college movie genre appears time and again in the oral histories, therapeutic notes and legal documents of Shy people and movement lawyers. The genre appears as a site of anxiety and distress, a factor in cases of Introvert hate crime and a cultural product that mitigates resistance operations. The American college movie inserts Shy peoples into taxonomies and binary labelling systems not of their choosing, and this is a source of rage, insecurity and distress.)

The plot: superficially attractive and popular female students, all called Heather, plus another girl, Veronica, embody the pinnacle of the Extrovert-Supremacist high school oligarchy. They engage in activities such as cheerleading, attend exclusive parties and date alpha males. The girls' regime of cronyism and cruelty involves acts of Introvert hate crime and inequality entrenchment. And yet, emerging from within the group as a proto-Aspergistan freedom fighter, Veronica notes in her private journal that she dreams of 'a world without *Heathers*... a world where I am free.'

It becomes impossible for Veronica to continue her collaboration with the Heathers' regime. At the start of the film she bullies a quiet fellow student, referred to by the Heathers as 'Dumptruck', but she soon develops empathy with the victim, as well as with such survivors as the Heathers label 'dweebettes', 'geeks' or 'pillowcases'. Thanks to her continued recourse to the Introvert self-training practice of diary keeping, Veronica has her political awakening. She initiates an Extrovert-abolitionist revolt against the *Heathers'* groupthink.

Veronica's subversion strategies include vomiting at an exclusive party, striking a humiliating blow to the Heathers' reputation. She proceeds to sabotage acts of Introvert hate crime, and refuses to comply with the alpha male's or jock's sexual pressures or listen to his macho boasting about sexual encounters that never happened. The maintenance of a diary prevails as a pillar of resistance for Veronica, and a device by which the film's plot can proceed: events are woven together with Veronica's introspective political demands and reflections.

Veronica continues her resistance operations in partnership with the elusive and enigmatic proto-Shy Radical, JD a new student at the college who dresses in a dark trench coat denoting his difference from the American football players and their Coca-Cola-red sportswear. Before long, Veronica and JD become a couple, and their arguments represent a set of wider political conversations about militancy and/or piecemeal change. They carry out a series of assassinations, first of the Heathers and later of the college jocks known as Brad, Ram and Kurt, covering them up by faking suicide notes in which the characters of the assassinated are rewritten with reference to the core Aspergistani values of 'depth', 'soul' and 'brain'.

Eventually Veronica turns her back on JD as the series of targeted assassinations continues. She renounces him as 'extreme', despairing that 'No one can stop JD . Not the FBI, not the CIA...' JD asserts that the high school embodies the values of the society and that society must begin again at Year Zero. When interrogated on the strategic assassination of college jocks, JD simply asks: 'What did they have to offer the world except date rape and AIDS jokes?'

The film is still debated in Shy Radical circles: given its absence of better alternatives or utopian horizons, does *Heathers* present a hopeful or hopeless vision? New Shy Radicals claim identification with both Veronica and JD with some even confessing to feeling heartbroken at the couple splitting and turning on each other. Others take the stance that Veronica represents the failures and state collaboration of the Introvert Rights Association. Does the revenge fantasy remain just a fantasy?

Towards the close of the film, JD attempts a guerrilla-style insurrection against the college building, planting a bomb during a cheerleading and sports rally. At the close of the film, following the insurrection's failure, JD asserts that 'the only place different social types can get along with each other is in heaven', and commits suicide by self-immolating.

Some Shy Radicals were disappointed in the ending of the film, as it draws a problematic distinction between the 'moderate' Introvert reformist Veronica, and the 'psycho'- pathological JD. Veronica comes out on top, despite having turned her back on overthrowing the system. Walking the high-school corridor in the final scenes, Veronica declares herself the 'new sheriff in town', by rejecting the judgements of the remaining Heather girl and snatching a red hairband. Much like a Western development NGO, she reaches out to the quiet 'Dumptruck' character by inviting her to watch movies and play croquet. Veronica declares that Extrovert-Supremacy is 'not my style'. But does she ever relinquish her power? Does it ever transfer to Dumptruck and other true Shy Radicals?

THE 'STUDIO INTROVERT' QUESTION

The Shy Radicals forum debated whether *Heathers* is an example of the downward spiral of Introvert identity into marketisation and commodification. The film is recognised as a landmark in Winona Ryder's career given her repeat casting thereafter as iconic 'outsider' and 'misfit': she appears in Tim Burton's *Beetlejuice* (1988) and *Edward Scissorhands* (1990), and continues along this trajectory throughout the 1990s with appearances in Jim Jarmusch's *Night on Earth* (1991), the Generation-x film *Reality Bites* (1994), before playing the glamorised psychiatric patient sectioned alongside Angelina Jolie in *Girl, Interrupted* (1999). Perhaps the highlight of Ryder's career is when she appears in a special episode of *The Simpsons* called 'Lisa's Rival': in this instance she is cast as a new friend to Shy Radical icon Lisa Simpson, exhibiting new levels of sensitivity and introversion.

Those in attendance at the debate were invited to write alternative endings to *Heathers*. How could it be made more progressive? How could it re-envision the society it presents as unchangeable? Research by the Introvert Studies Association has revealed that the original ending had a twist: the reformist Veronica eventually engages in her own suicide bombing of the school. Pressure by McCarthyite Hollywood studio executives forced this conclusion to be left on the cutting-room floor. The Shy Radicals' us delegation has since pressurised the film industry into reissuing a DVD boxset with the additional suicide bombing included. A sequel for the film was also rumoured but was never made.

Further notes: In 2010, the next wave of the Introfada was triggered by the announcement that *Heathers* would be produced as a musical for Broadway. The news was met with horror: song titles included 'Seventeen', 'Candy Store' and 'Mean Girls' and the glossy chick-lit-style marketing was deemed to be abhorrent, giving rise to further currents of protest across the Shy International. The musical was restaged internationally in London's West End and beyond. The Shy Radicals' US delegation unsuccessfully initiated a boycott. Later, methods of sabotage were discussed but not enacted. The Introvert Rights Association suggested that a network of lobbying would suffice. In August 2014, when at last *Heathers: The Musical* ceased to be performed, its death was celebrated internationally through academic symposia and silent vigils.

Behind the Candelabra (2013)
Director: Steven Soderbergh.
USA.
118 mins.

The Liberace biopic *Behind the Candelabra* was screened at a number of Shy Radical student societies. It later emerged that the screenings were being used to help the students understand the intersection of the Enemy, where race, class and extrovert-supremacy meet. This elite razzmatazz decadence could also be found in the new generation of American college TV series: Beverly Hills 90210, the 'cribs' of MTV, the swimming pools blocs of Israeli settlements, the mansion of popular girl Cher in *Clueless* and settler-colonialism in North Africa.

At first students watched the scenes of the mansion where black chambermaids serve with sparse dialogue. The students were encouraged to view the film from the perspective of this maid rather than those with their names in lights. Here Liberace serves as European Roman emperor, Pharaoh and Marie Antoinette-styled pre-revolutionary French aristocrat: complete with classical sculptures, chandeliers, Jacuzzis, ballrooms and foot soldiers. Above, the extrovert-supremacism icon tried to change the nature of the candle as introvert light to extrovert light by propping them in diamond studded candelabra. During his performance the boogie-woogie is upped in tempo to sixteen beats to a bar, anticipating the orthodoxy of the total positivity trance club. In one line, he exclaims: 'Black piano, black tuxedo, who is going to see me in this giant calm shell?' revealing the anti-introvert contempt, leading to generations of Introvert Hate crime. Attempts at pink washing this extrovert-supremacism have been rejected by Shy Radical student delegations with a split in the student LGBTQI society.

The students also studied and analysed archives of Liberace's TV appearances. His extremist permanent smile, glittery jackets and opulent clothing were particularly shocking and frightening to some audience members. One of these items consisted of a 16 ft. long virgin fox coat. Items of his clothing were also made with $100, 000 of mined diamonds. This lead to new forms of high sensitivity certification being considered for the TV shows.

The Battle of Algiers (1966)
Director: Gillo Pontecorvo.
Italy/Algeria.
121 minutes.

The Battle of Algiers has been deemed as the landmark anti-colonial film, used as a training tool for the PLO, Black Panthers and IRA, as well as by the US Army as a training tool for defeating insurgents in the 2003 Iraq War and by Argentinian intelligence during the Dirty War. The film was banned in France from 1965 until 1970 on national security grounds.

The screenplay is based on a memoir of FLN guerrilla leader Saadi Yucef. Despite its misreading through an Extrovert Supremacist lens, and despite a plethora of academic commentary, it is clear that this film is really about oppressed Shy people striking back. The film is a proto-Introfada film, showing the guerrilla army of wallflowers lurking in the corners and the shadows. During certain explosive, panic-stricken scenes, the urban guerrilla army expresses a certain disdain towards nightclubs.

The central protagonist, Ali La Pointe, an Algerian native turned guerrilla fighter, has also been misread by earlier generations as a victim of colonial underdevelopment due to his sparse dialogue throughout the film. It is very clear, from an Introvert Studies perspective, that his minimal speech is not simply due to illiteracy but because he is, in fact, really shy.

In an early scene in the film he is tripped up by brash French colonial settlers in one of the earliest instances of Introvert hate crime to be documented on the cinematic screen. His humiliation, echoing the playground bully of the introvert-class, forms a core part of his radicalisation. The film is also used as a training video to new recruits to devise strategy to new recruits to the Aspergistan cause. The opening scene starts with a torture scene, with a silent gaunt man surrounded by a gang of chauvinist French Colonial soldiers – attempting to pressure him into conviviality. 'Couldn't you have talked sooner?' spits out one of the soldiers. It emerges that the torture is being carried out in a bid to make the man talk. He remains silent. The ethical question of using torture to break a quiet sensibility remains for future generations, where such tactics are still in widespread use under the War on Terror by Extrovert-supremacist security state.

'We must isolate and destroy them' commands the French Colonial general to his army. And here we realise why they lose. Of course, due to the pitfalls of extrovert-normativity, he didn't realise that for introvert a period of isolation means to be recharged. And so, one day, the colonised will finally win the battle and national liberation. We shall overcome, towards the inevitable Aspergistan homeland.

EIGHT

CRISIS VOICES ORAL HISTORY PROJECT

The Introvert Rights Association's Crisis Voices was an oral history project conceived during Introvert History Month. The project documents the local Introvert Crisis Centres, funded by the state, local councils and lottery funding, set up to protect those who were seeking shelter and escape from Extrovert harassment and house party households. The centres were opened as an extension of the Introvert Youth Helpline, again set up with the same stakeholders and funders. The project received diversity award mental health funding and was administered by the Introvert Rights Association, shortly before their split and internal implosion, leading to their breakaway to the Shy Radical movement. The defection towards a new, more challenging form of political representation was consolidated at this point.

The recordings were distributed in schools, colleges and community centres as a means to create 'social cohesion' and to foster 'diversity, dialogue and peace'. It later emerged through a whistle-blower that these recordings were not the originals; they had been heavily censored internally, by the Introvert Rights Association, following concerns that its funding might be affected by the dissemination of 'subversive', 'radical' and 'separatist' views. The tapes were leaked to the Shy Radicals Underground, who now use the Shy Radicals website for the presentation of the full transcripts. A selection of transcripts, containing the words of staff and clients at the domestic centres, is presented here as a mosaic of despair, containing within it the uncensored voices of some of the most troubled participants.

INTERVIEW WITH STAFF MEMBER NURSE JENNA: CATALOGUE NO.1/24507AB

INTERVIEWER: TELL ME WHEN YOU FIRST SET UP THIS CENTRE?

NURSE JENNA: We were supposed to set up therapeutic environments, which we did and which we maintained as places where Introverts could feel safe, at home, free. Everything was adapted–

space and time for rejuvenation, investigation and research. Book-shelves stretched as far as the eye could see, a garden with a tran-quil placid lake, cosy and intimate spaces inside where you could drink mint tea, camomile tea, lemon and ginger tea, exotic teas, and with honey instead of sugar. The lighting was made to re-semble evening desk-light – perfect for contemplation. It was-somewhere for Introverts to come and recharge their batteries.

Some of the Introverts became research subjects, and we could use this research to examine other forms of pathological social withdrawal, as was taking place in Japan for example. We could reintegrate our clients with healthy, happy, positive, outgoing people. Not all of them accepted our rehabilitation methods… I asked why they were here then. Sometimes I told them to go home if they didn't want to be part of the programme. I know I shouldn't have. Or should I?

One day a light bulb malfunctioned. And it started flashing and flashing and flashing, non-stop. It was like a strobe light in one of them discos. I remember screams throughout the night: 'TRENDY CLUB! TRENDY CLUB!' It created a panic in the Introvert household. We were on full staff alert. We had an emergency. Some of the inmates even ran to the exits. Or threw themselves out of windows. The less said about that the better.

Emergency aside, no one wanted to leave. We had readmissions and our resources were overstretched. The problem was when the Introvert client left the centre, and went into the so-called real world, they would always relapse. They saw a drop in their self-esteem, to the point of self-loathing. Just walking along the street or watching TV would create a depressive slump and the feeling of being unwanted, disposable, with the familiar symp-toms of withdrawal, sleeping all day, etc. Their working environ-ments were often unsuitable: office parties, the demand to fake enthusiasm to sell products. They would want to escape again, back to us. I'd say 'Sorry, honey, we don't have room to shelter you tonight.' The therapeutic environment could only provide tempo-rary relief. We were faced with a crisis we couldn't hope to solve.

**INTERVIEW WITH STAFF MEMBER NURSE SEAN:
CATALOGUE NO. 7/28507TB**

Not all the Introvert clients trusted me. I was not one of them, they said. I mean I like a drink. I like a laugh. I don't take myself too seriously.

**INTERVIEW WITH ANONYMOUS INTROVERT CLIENT:
CATALOGUE NO. 18/99837JK**

They told me if I was unhappy, I could write to my MP to complain about Extrovert-Supremacy...

**INTERVIEW WITH ANONYMOUS INTROVERT CLIENT:
CATALOGUE NO. 15/50766YC**

Being intelligent and sensitive gets you nowhere in life... and some of us grew up on our own myths that there would be some reward somewhere. I was brainwashed by those films like *Dead Poets Society* – they led me to believe that there was some higher, more authentic value to be found in actually enjoying the literary canon; a reward at the end of the storm.And then there were books like *The Catcher in the Rye*... I remember as a teenager I used to call myself after the protagonist Holden Caulfield – that was my name in internet chat rooms to indicate that I was that sensitive guy, suffering in a phony world. I thought to myself, I suffered in the earlier stages of life... But there would be some reward at the end... wouldn't there? Otherwise what was the value of rebellion? Where was the exit? Was I condemned to a loop of humiliation? I reached the end of my tether asking these questions. It was a handful of dust. Just despair.

I was unemployed for a very long time. I ceased to remember what it was like to work. My adviser forced me to take on the roles of tourist rep, salesman and charity street recruiter. I put it off as long as I could; I spent my teens and twenties avoiding the kind of work they tried to give me. I couldn't handle the retail or sales sector. I couldn't do telephone marketing. I really couldn't. I didn't fit their conception of this 'everyone' who purportedly could do these jobs...

I couldn't escape it. Eventually I was made to stand in the middle of the street, assaulting passersby for some NGO I didn't care for, as part of the new Workfare reforms. I realised that even those who displayed enthusiasm didn't care. But they could pull up a skilled fake energy they got from being 'outgoing', whereas I couldn't hide my real feelings of disillusionment and contempt. I felt so manipulative, I couldn't do it. Eventually I was sacked. It happened again. Same pattern. Smile. Have a nice day! Couldn't manage it. Stiff gestures showed themselves. They were inbuilt in my limbs. I was sacked. I felt happier in an administrative job, in a closed cubicle, but then came the office parties of the Christmas season. I started. I was sacked. I started... Sometimes it would go on for years. I went into a downward spiral. I was told I didn't qualify for a disability. I wasn't sure I was disabled. In the end, I wound up here.

Sometimes I wouldn't even get a job. I wouldn't even get short-listed for an interview. I found that if there were two sets of people with identical qualifications, in each and every case, the Extrovert would come first. It was the same in many other instances, people like us would be marooned and rejected. The world was plastic, inflexible, candyfloss, artificial. We couldn't cope in such a world.

I used to sleep all day and spend seven hours a day on Facebook. Doner kebabs weren't good for me but they made me feel good. And motivated me to wake up in the afternoon. Some of the other... Residents? Inmates? Clients? Patients? Participants? They silently formed a faction within the centre. They didn't accept what the staff told them. They started to see me as a betrayer; doner kebabs were 'post-nightclub intake'. There would be serious debates about my eating habits in the house, and they'd go on until the midnight hours as if they were a serious matter, like the resolution of war and peace. The longest debate took place at the end of a Friday night binge. There were new rules being set. They said they would organise. And that was off-limits to me. Their organising proved that I wasn't one of them and that I didn't belong. They took it too seriously. It was like being vegan or lactose intolerant. I had to check every ingredient in the food I wanted to consume to see if it was Extrovert. I called them... *inmates*... I even then called them fascists. Then I realised they were the good guys, part of the resistance and that I wanted to join the struggle.

INTERVIEW WITH ANONYMOUS INTROVERT CLIENT: CATALOGUE NO.22/985071O

[An artist, he has chosen to remain anonymous for what he says is a political reason. He has not participated in the art world for a number of years.]

I first got into art because I did not like football at school in the playground. Being in a gallery was one place I could experience a certain type of silence. I keep scrapbooks of cuttings and ideas and collections. I like the texture of things, getting lost in abstract patterns. The sombre abstract of a low-lit painting by Rothko: low lighting was a condition he set and demanded for the gallery. You had to admire that. There was a pleasure, too, in the simple, gradual drying of watercolours and oil. Minimal abstraction, I could invest that with wonder. It made me feel at home. I had to learn the hard way that the art world, with its fast-paced trends and works made by quiet fabricators and assistants for Extrovert artists, wasn't the place for people like me. It was hard. And now I'm here... at the Introvert Crisis Centre.

Private views, parties, press and patrons make the art world go round. I'd been enthused about delving into the history of art and the archive, about attending art theory seminars. When I was at university I thought that it was a matter of getting a first-class degree. I was so naive.

It hurt me the most when my application was rejected for

a front-of-house role at the central cultural quarter at the South-bank Centre which houses the Royal Festival Hall, Poetry Library, Hayward Gallery, Purcell Room, all my favourite places, all my good memories. Despite spending half my teens wandering from galleries to poetry evenings to reference libraries, I was rejected before I got to interview. Twice. I could only conclude that they didn't like my personality. And yet, on reflection, after withdrawing to the slump of my bed, I thought about it. What was this customer service I couldn't do? I am a person who actually uses all these cultural venues yet I was being told by the big Extrovert, with a smile so fake I was certain her face would crack, that I could not be allowed to be a service to people like... myself... I mean I was being prohibited from performing customer service in my own world... why did the gatekeepers not let me in? Who was Mr Customer Service? Customer Service wanted me written out of existence.

Or maybe it was worse in the 1990s. I took my first trip to Paris. I went to the Palais de Tokyo. It was all open spaces, like a factory they claimed though I didn't understand how. I just liked how it was open until midnight at the time. I wished that every-where could be like that, including in London. But the Palais de Tokyo merged its openness with a certain culture of the neon nightclub. When I realised what was going on I felt that something sacred was being trampled over, spectacularised. At the same time, a new kind of art was being globalised. They called it 'relational aesthetics'. Rirkrit Tiravanija's food parties, demanding that everyone partake in eating curry in the gallery, were being hailed as a new type of art. Coercive social interaction sponsored by Hugo Boss was the crux of this art. This was supposed to be emancipatory? When I listened to the lectures, it all turned out to be false, a facile mimicry of participatory democracy.

Contemporary art reached the public through the atten-tion-grabbing sensationalism of the tabloids. The broadsheets were just as stupid. A small sanctuary of sense could be found in the academic journals. But something was missing even there: the academic texts hinted at wonder and feeling, gave a sense of investigation. But all the love and inspiration was lost to excessive referencing, the over-professionalism of it all. The journals became a false refuge for me when I realised that the academics were just doing their jobs. Where else could a sanctuary be found in present day society?

State funding for arts organisations was in the name of participation and so-called 'access'. But the bureaucratic funding forms were never able to capture what I understood access to be: something that could never be quantified, an inner richness of experience. We had to fill in forms to assess our performance indicators. The onus was always placed on numbers of people or 'audience figures', and demographic categories were key. We needed an entire new language, an entirely new form of public accountability to assess the inner richness that our institutions could provide. What was really happening to people on the inside? What was really enriching about their engagement? The language of spirituality was a forgotten shore, maybe.

The royal families of Qatar and Saudi Arabia sponsored this art world, and it profited them in turn. Everyone wanted a piece of the Qatari pie. Damien Hirst was funded by royal and oil money. I went to the Middle East in the hope that I would find something different. It was a culture shock. But mostly because my experience of it was the same as my experience of London. At the opening party of some biennale, fifty-year-old academics were behaving like decadent partygoers. It was so depressing. My stomach was a pit of despair. Why was I still in this world?

I got to thinking that my space had been colonised. There were artists who made art. And there were fashionistas who made fashions. Art was Palestine. Fashion was Israel, being colonised and cleansed.

I wasn't happy with the way things were and the way things were going. I was told there were official procedures for dealing with grievances and a complaints process in the institution. And beyond that the local council, and above the police, the courts, the law, the parliament, even up to the United Nations. It was like a moving train and I wanted to hit the brakes. And when I started at the lowest level, voicing my concerns to the staff, they treated me differently.

INTERVIEW WITH INTROVERT CLIENT JAMIE X: CATALOGUE NO.3/282340B

[Jamie x, now known as Azadi following his conversion to Islam, has since described himself as feeling lost.]

I thought that Islam was the last remaining bulwark against the forces of Extrovert-Supremacism. I was wrong, very wrong. Any inner-city manifestation of Islam will testify to this, from the Paris suburbs to West Yorkshire's Bradistan; all the 'boyz n the hood' posturing as Muslim 'bad boy' youth. Bad spoken word and slam poetry, just to go on their YouTube vanity channels, gesturing hands waving their 'street' attitude in your face. There's no shielding yourself from all this. Global evangelical TV superstars like Dr Zakir Naik, the *Boyz II Men* nasheeds produced like super clean smooth RnB, the celebrity narcissism of evangelical Dawah preachers across digital cable channels worldwide... seeing the hijabi girls in the shopping centres of Westfield in full knowledge of who it was funding their avowed Zionist enemy through its ownership by a former Israeli commando. And these macho younger guys like the Muslim Debate Initiatives on the speaker circuits of the Friday khutabs, student Islamic Societies that wanted to challenge everyone who opposed them to a debate... I had been brought up on bookish and mild-mannered English gentleman Sufism; the words of the Cambridge-based scholar and interfaith activity leader T. J. Winter (Shaykh Abdal Hakim Murad); and the writings of Martin Lings (Abu Bakr Siraj ad-Din), author of the beautifully referenced biography of the Prophet Muhammad. Urban Islam came as a shock to my system; street Dawah, charity fundraisers only undertaking religious conversion

– pitting 'Socialism vs Islam', 'Atheism vs Islam' and uploading their successes online – appeared in stark contrast to all that I'd come to know and admire. Then there were Ali and Mo – your standard street-corner Asian boy munching away in the Halal Fried Chicken shop, imagining they were in the Bronx – with their big fat Nike Air trainers, latest smart phone and their sports car aspirations. Why was it all so in sync with capitalism? Maybe it wasn't the true Islam. I don't know.

I turned atheist at first. I used to drink. I used to drink alcohol a lot. Because I was painfully shy, and alcohol made me like them – allowed me to more closely resemble and just about tolerate the party people. Although I hated myself, I no longer had to be shy when I was drinking. Thanks to the so-called social lubricant, I could imitate them. Sometimes I wouldn't even remember what I was saying. And then I realised, that drinking for a Shy person is a form of self-hating, consisting of fooling yourself into thinking that you could only be free if you were imitating them. What kind of liberation was that? You could only be tolerated if you were one of them, one of the gregarious, loudmouthed and brash and yet perversely more socially acceptable people. The prevailing order of things allowed these people to command attention, to be the 'life' and the 'soul'. So now, I don't drink anymore. Tea has replaced beer. People put it down to my conversion to Islam. But that wasn't it: now, as a matter of pride and principle, I don't drink. I am myself. I am truly free; I have a freedom of selfhood and a sense of pride. Shy people who drink hate themselves and hate their people. They become traitors in spite of themselves. I once wrote: 'Extrovert-Supremacism systematically verifies itself when the slave can only break free by imitating the master: by denying his own reality.'

Have you seen the Woody Allen film *Play It Again, Sam?* It features Woody Allen as a neurotic sensitive case and he sees apparitions of Humphrey Bogart who offers him advice like a mentor. I imagine myself in a parallel scenario, only with Ayatollah Khomeini in the role of counsellor instead of Humphrey Bogart. Every time I was at a horrible private view, staring at my feet, I would imagine an apparition of Imam Khomeini – he would console me with his cautions against those decadent Westerners. He would strike them off.

INTERVIEW WITH INTROVERT CLIENT KURT WILLIAMS: CATALOGUE NO.92/22227TB

[Kurt Williams had escaped from a university in the North of England, whilst in the middle of a PhD, to an Introvert Rights Association household domestic centre. He was later thrown out of the centre and made homeless after literature from Shy Radicals political prisoners was found his room. His whereabouts remain unknown. Rumours have it that he joined a Shy Radical Underground cell. An intricate drawing of the Aspergistan flag motif '...' etched secretly over several nights on the windowpane of the central London Introvert Crisis Centre was thought to be of his doing. None of the attempts at gathering forensic evidence have helped locate his hiding place.]

When I went to school I was bullied. I was unhappy. I found humiliation in the playground. I was unhappy in class. I was picked on. They saw me as easy prey. I was vulnerable and open to attack. There was nothing about my demeanour that said 'don't f——with me'. When I moved up from primary to secondary school, then from college to university, I felt a lot better. Or so I thought. I thought of education as a filtering process. The higher you get up, the more finely those bullying elements get filtered out.

Other Black and Asian kids, Muslims, Hindus, Christians, Sikhs, would bully me for being too quiet. I remember the TV series Baywatch with Pamela Anderson, its celebrity stars were popular when I was a kid, except for the flat-chested woman who the Pakistani kids referred to as my girlfriend. So much for their solemnity. Who could make things better for me?

It should be noted that I experienced a similar sense of betrayal when my admiration for the work of Sylvia Plath – *The Bell Jar* with the early cover design filled with abstract swirling spirals – was overtaken by the remarketing of her as 'chick lit', and my resigned discovery that the chick lit version more accurately reflected her persona in real life. I'd assumed that her beauty was that of the interior world of Ariel and Thumb. But in fact she valued the other world, and suffered for it. And it was taken on exclusively by campus feminists as a woman's cause. But they didn't consider why it connected with us too as alienated men. It was a trauma and a betrayal seeing this. It was difficult. I found other writers I liked such as Ann Quin, an experimental author largely forgotten about these days, and Anna Kavan. I wouldn't let them be claimed exclusively as a women's cause too. I remember Doris Lessing being claimed by all sorts of people she didn't agree with before she turned to Sufism. Then there were distinguished academics in fields like anthropology – one favourite of mine was Saba Mahmood. Saba wrote some anthropological work in Egypt about the political nature of listening in the mosque network. She questioned the very nature of Liberal representation through identifying agency in women committed to Islamist causes – how they used the Quran as a constitution to level themselves up. I realised then there were other ways of being empowered. I realised what I had been made to believe about cloaked-up women as docile and submissive people was a lie. This had wider implications. Was the model on the advertising billboard really empowered? Visibility didn't equal power.

I felt betrayed when I grew up and observed the lifestyles of the academics. Academics with engagements in Ibiza, their pictures in my face on Instagram, their self-promotional tweets filling my timeline. They were just into the parties and shallow forms of competition and nepotism, sporting Jimmy Choo and Marc Jacobs' bags, Maison Martin Margiela sneakers that they described as 'art-world standard issue'. They were so utterly exhibitionist. At first I felt embarrassed. I felt betrayed. It hurt me. I thought there was nowhere left to turn. There was even a cultural studies book called Club Cultures: Music, Media and Subcultural Capital, which I was so eager to read, assuming that it would be a reassuringly aloof academic takedown of clubbing culture, penned using an arcane and vengeful critical lexicon... I confess that was my original motivation for getting into academia... a quiet world of revenge fantasy... but... but [sobs]. The argument was that clubbing was emancipatory... long silence]. Academia was supposed to be my escape and here it was endorsing my idea of hell, with peer reviews by Stuart Hall and the like. Academia was supposed to be the better alternative but even lecturing these days was like performing on a stage.

INTERVIEW WITH ANONYMOUS INTROVERT CLIENT: CATALOGUE NO. 44/44507TC

[A young woman, at the time of the interview she had recently been engaged to be married.]

I ran out of my wedding. I like the idea of marriage. But the wedding... It was too much. Most weddings are so showy, with sequins, a flowing headdress, decadence and extravagance: too much. Earlier in my life I thought that Asian weddings were more dignified than white peoples' wedding. There were no aunties and uncles disco-dancing. But the Asian weddings are the ultimate worst, competing in flashiness and showiness with the big fat Greek wedding, the big Punjabi wedding. Another hell for me that made me run away, and keep running, until I found shelter here: in the Introvert Crisis Centre.

I haven't been in touch with my husband since. I wasn't charmed or attracted by Extrovert alpha men but I thought they could protect me. But I found though that 'protection' can constitute a form of abuse. When we are forced into protective environments, not all of us can enjoy them. We can't celebrate. I know people, including myself, who delayed marriage in order to avoid the brashness and dishonesty of the 'celebration', the 'special day'. But we never speak honestly about it, to avoid ruining the specialness of the ceremony for everyone else.

But the truth is there and it's undeniable: we hate it.

I used to think that you couldn't escape this. You're a young woman they said, you should be elated by the prospect of your wedding day, one of the best days of your life. I craved middle age and no longer having to care, sailing past the supposed sanctuary of motherhood and becoming a 'yummy mummy', a social category designed by the people at the top of the heteronormative social order to make us feel self-conscious and depressed about our bodies. Already depressed, I joined a dating website for a week to consider the alternatives. But the problems of in-person encounters were simply reflected back at me there, in photos given to showiness. People posing in places I didn't enjoy. I remembered it being different on the internet; I used to meet others who were more like me. Now I had to search harder for them, eventually finding communities who didn't accept the central authority and who introduced me to new concepts. They told me what 'Extrovert-Supremacism' was, and it all made sense. They opened my eyes...

The environment was home. It was like an umbrella, a shelter. But we couldn't shake an awareness of the outside. We all had scars, we all had chains. We knew that the Crisis Centre was only providing temporary relief from the ongoing assault of Extrovert-Supremacism. We couldn't stay under this umbrella forever. We wanted shelter but we needed to break out... to change the outside. So we began to think of the Introvert Crisis Centre as our training ground.

The nature of Extrovert-Supremacism was first explained to me through the children's cartoon Teenage Mutant Ninja Turtles. There was Michelangelo, the Ninja Turtle with an addiction to pizza and a compulsion to say the word 'Cowabunga!', based on a 'surfer dude' style Extrovert-Supremacist. Splinter, on the other hand, was one of us: the series' rat leader was an Introvert master of self-discipline and fluent in the art of ancient Japanese lore and medi-tation. The Ninja Turtle Leonardo was also one of us: much more cautious than Michaelangelo, and with an intelligent grasp of the katana sword.

The influence of Michaelangelo dominated nonetheless: I saw the triumph of his idiocy over the superior intellect of his Ninja peers and leader as a pattern replicated throughout the entire structure of children's television. Children's TV presenters were the worst. I remember wanting, as a child, to be left alone to be absorbed in my crayon and chalk drawings. But the television was always on, and the TV presenter, with his positive, swirling curly eyes and big overenthusiastic voice would come over and interrupt me and my train of thought. These interrupting people haunted me into my adult life: they were always at an advantage in the world of jobs, living and sustaining the assumption that all of us want to be addressed in a booming voice. They mistake loudness for having a personality. It is my idea of hell to be stuck in a room with people like that. The room becomes a party. The schoolroom inherits this atmosphere too, because schoolteachers follow the logic of the children's TV presenter. It's truly contagious: even nursery staff and nannies tend towards flashiness and overenthusiasm. Eventually, it is widely assumed that the children's TV presenter type is the only type of person capable of caring for kids. Some adoption agencies give preferential treatment to this type. The logic spreads like a virus and this is how it comes to dominate the world. It is true that a few of the university professors and academics are more like our people, bookish and Introvert. But with exposure to Extrovert-Supremacism in the early stages of childhood, pre-primary school, more and more of us are growing up scarred and conditioned.

INTERVIEW WITH ANONYMOUS STAFF MEMBER: CATALOGUE NO.37/28557HB

Some of the long-term clients started to invent new rules for the institution. They didn't accept our authority as staff. They didn't accept that we were their patrons. They didn't follow the step-by-step programme so carefully devised for their benefit. They rejected the assertiveness life skills training we provided.

One of the new rules consisted of banning the use of the 'N-word'. At first, I thought they were referring to banning derogatory references to Black people. But they said that of course that reference was already banned and in this instance they were talking about some of the new clients' self-identification as 'nerds'. A few of the older clients said the word 'nerd' brought back very painful memories for them: of feeling low, excluded, shut out. They said to use it would make the speaker complicit in something they called 'Introvert hate crime', which upheld 'the system'. And yet these terms did not appear in our handbooks. Our staff training had equipped us with all kinds of strategies for dealing with troubled conversations. But it hadn't prepared us for this. The 'N-word' always promoted an inferiority complex, they said. So they set rules with the aim of engaging with the Crisis Centre's programme on their own terms.

INTERVIEW WITH ANONYMOUS INTROVERT CLIENT: CATALOGUE NO. 90/28117TJ

Why in most scenarios do these loudmouth people just naturally assume they are in charge? The new rules we set for ourselves in the safe house taught me: don't take it. The institution was not our shelter: it made us dependent. We were more than just problem-cases.

REPORT FROM THE
INVERNESS DELEGATION

During the run-up to the Scottish independence referendum, we were not feeling the unity of either YES or NO. At this decisive moment in history, we felt great unease and concern at the feel-good electioneering of the SNP campaign, the parades, the patriotism, chauvinism, fireworks bravado, the Highland Games, the *Braveheart*-style hype, and other such antics. It made us feel a wee bit anxious… and it was not just the break away from England and Wales that we feared. Some of us didn't feel included in the Scottish nation – the ceremonial aspect simply was not representative of the way we identified with the world.

We dissented from the party line of all existing progressive gatherings and Scottish nationalist parties and the YES campaign itself. At first, we created a splinter group and held regular meetings in Inverness at Leakey's, one of the last independent bookshops in the city. Originally a Gaelic church, the place had an open log fire and a cafe serving homemade food. It was an original Shy Radical resistance hub: its clientele were those who'd grown disaffected by the identikit cities that locations such as Glasgow were turning into. They would come along, bemoaning the fact that every high street was now geared towards Extrovert-Supremacism. The meeting group occupied Leakey's Bookshop on the weekends, laying the foundations for a campaign for twenty-four-hour access to bookshops. It wasn't about buying more. It was about having somewhere to inhabit. We needed bookshops to be open at all times so that we had somewhere to feel at home, to ruminate away from Scotland's so-called 'working class' drinking culture. We didn't recognise or relate to Irvine Welsh's depictions of the Scottish working class in novels like *Trainspotting*, *Filth*, *Porno* or *Ecstasy*, all of them repetitious of each other, with their descriptions of getting 'goosed', 'blootered', 'oot yer tree', 'oot yer tits', 'slooshed', 'rubbered', 'minced', 'reakin', 'trollied', 'sloozled', 'mad wae it', and 'floored' on a night out. That was not our language. Night was a long walk into the soul. We were not part of that nation, any more than we were part of a kilt-wearing, bagpipe-playing culture, especially when the kilts were made for the catwalk and the tartan-chic magazine shoots. Ane leid is nivver eneuch, they say here, one language is never enough. What would that really mean after independence? As Scotland sought to remain part of the European Union after the Brexit vote, we looked at Inverness entering the political federation of Aspergistan, to become part of that autonomous federal union.

What did we treasure about Scotland? After Leakey's in Inverness, Beauly was beautiful – bleak, quiet and peaceful. It was possible to enjoy the slow pleasure of trout-fishing there, and of long, gentle walks. Then there was Durness, which had gorgeous stretches of empty sandy beaches whose character we wanted to preserve: They were the opposite of tourist-trap beaches such as those of Ibiza and Brighton, which bred hot-air hedonism. And Durness's Smoo Cave, with its internal waterfall, was unique, deep and beautiful, with archaeological digs revealing layers of Norse and Neolithic history. Another beautiful, peaceful place in Scotland, for mossy rocks, castle ruins, placid, undisturbed rock pools: the Fairy Pools on the Isle of Skye. The new nationalist government wanted to encourage the wrong type of tourism in such places – income-generating and socially regenerating (if environmentally destructive) gentrifying tourism. We, as an international cell and delegation of Aspergistan, offered to protect the Smoo Cave and Fairy Pools by any means necessary.

Throughout history, nationalist struggles always created some sort of homage to ageless unspoilt rural landscapes…You see that in the opening rolling aerial shots of *Braveheart*, over the Highlands… We don't want a homage. We want the real thing, in Scotland and in locations inhabited by Shy groups worldwide. We protect the homeland for long walks and peaks of solitary reverie.

We felt a need to retreat to rural Scotland to recharge, away from it all, before it engulfed us, wandering among the forgotten Manx and Gaelic dialects of the Inner Hebrides archipelago. We too felt our existence threatened. Around a log-fire, we listened to the post-rock band Mogwai's albums – *Government Commissions*, the soundtracks for *Zidane*, *The Fountain*, *Les Revenents*. In their slowness and abstraction, and with Mogwai's wordless, hushed singing, it felt like a set of hymns for an alternative nation.

TEN

RUPTURES IN THE EXTROVERT WORLD ORDER: BREAKING INTROFADA STRUGGLE

THE BALKANS: SEVDAH VERSUS TURBO-FOLK

SARAJEVO, BOSNIA: The ethnic and religious divisions that formed in the wars in the break-up of the former Yugoslavia took on a new shape. No longer was one nominally an Orthodox Serb, a Muslim Bosniak or Catholic Croat. Identity and territory were shaped by a new sensibility. This needed to be marked in other ways from the Dayton Accords peace agreement, which cemented the ethno-religious divisions yet further. This broke out into the Balkan Introfada...

Thumping, pumping and humping... Turbo-folk originates in Serbia. A mash-up of speeded-up Balkan fiddler folk with upbeat techno-pop rhythms. Our Sarajevo delegation designated this genre as 'music for looking, not listening'. Videos appear very similar to other genres of globalised club, FHM lifestyle magazines and R'n'B music. Open-top sports cars, silicone, Barbie-doll women. Popular turbo-folk hits include 'Sexy Businessman', 'Belgrade Boys or Selfie', 'Suck this, Bosniak', 'Turn Me On, Turn Me Off', 'Gotta Twerk, Twerk, Work, Work' and 'Busty Party Hey Hey'.

Turbo-folk singers compared themselves to commanders with references to borders, pride. Serb national heroes litter songs, leading some to describe the genre as 'porno-nationalism'. Some singers went further and served on the frontline of the military occupation, always proud of their contribution to the Greater Serbia war effort. The state during Tito's unified communist Yugoslavia refused to financially support the genre of music due to its kitschy, tacky and commercial formula.

The music served as a soundtrack to the Bosnian genocide during the very worst incidents of mass rape, and the destruction of Ottoman heritage. Paramilitary commanders such as the notorious Željko 'Arkan' Ražnatović married turbo-folk star Ceca Veličković in a televised public ceremony. In the Milosevic/post-war era, turbo-folk has often been the music of the mafia economy. Ceca was later put under house arrest for embezzlement and for hiding a cache of assault rifles in her basement.

The genre further spread into Greece, Albania and Russia. The conspiracy behind the *Gangnam Style* crash led by Amy Littlewood (before her incarceration) discussed the possibility of crashing turbo-folk TV. stations such as Pink TV. The overlapping wave of Gangnam V-pop, turbo-folk and formulaic Western pop blurred more and more into each other as an ultra-refined form of Extrovert blandness.

Sevdah music is a national folk tradition, hailing from Bosnia. It is characterised by melancholic and yearning vocals – sometimes described as the Bosnian blues. Some see the Sevdah as continuing the Ottoman traditions. There is no exact translation in English. Its origins come the Arabic word *sawda* meaning 'black bile' – or 'melancholy' – from the times when it was believed that the human psychological make-up was attributable to the balance of the four humours.

The appeal of sevdah music extended beyond Sarajevo. It also had a following in Serbia and the Bosnian-Serb entity Republica Sprska, transcending religious, ethnic and military divides. Beyond the Balkans, a transnational alliance between the Fado Division in Lisbon and the Sevdah delegation to bolster international solidarity. Transitional political parties sprung up after the war such as Sevdah Democratic Action (SDA).

Nothing captures the essence of the struggle more than the dichotomy of the two genres: Sevdah (the Friend), turbo-folk (the Enemy). Just listen. Can those two genres really belong to the same tribe, life-world, nation, peoples? There the Friend-Enemy political distinction naturally plays itself out.

SHY RADICALS VERSUS EUROPEAN STATE SECULARISM

ISTANBUL, TURKEY: EU boundaries were guarded to prevent the flow of Shy people into the state. With the ascendancy of the AKP Islamist party, orders of the disciples of Rumi and Sufi were opened up again. Such practices had been repressed in the name of Kemal Ataturk's reforms. They were deemed by the dominant

European power Germany of becoming too popular, and were flowing westward. The Berlin club culture has been threatened and replaced with a Sufi order in residency, whirling dervishes chanting repetitive praises in the names of God. Would this create a new Europe vulnerable to Islamic Extrovert-Supremacism?

PARIS, FRANCE: The Shy Radicals movement is under state repression. The French authorities accuse the movement of violating the state conception of secularism known as *laïcité*. It is alleged that their excessive use of silence is an attempt to insert religion into the public sphere.

Members of the Paris delegation had earlier spent time sitting in silence in the cathedrals of Paris. These solemn silences were an escape from the tourist traps and bustle of the shopping districts. The movement aspires to create a public order that resembles a monastic order. Accusations from the authorities followed, as the radicals formed a conspiracy to recreate those silences within and without the cathedral dome. The interior of Notre Dame was fast turning into a tourist spectacle with flashing cameras everywhere. The Eurostar train, the visits to Calais...

Tourists marvel at the size and spectacle of the Eiffel Tower. But marvellous is the intricate mathematical engineering that sustains its erection. On special national occasions, the Mayor of Paris lights up the entire tower like a Christmas tree – a bright *tricolore* beaming across the city. But whose *liberté, égalité, fraternité?* Whither *la République indivisible*?

A further complication ensued when portraits of Marie Antoinette started to go missing from state museums. Suspects were immediately rounded up from the Shy Radicals delegation in dawn police raids.

Maoist French philosophers have also come out in support by writing a polemic in Le Monde. 'Behind the ban, is fear.' An extract from the piece: 'The destabilising effect of silence. That is something that brings about real self-examination. Our so-called leaders don't want to come face to face with themselves.

Otherwise the terror of their own self-doubt would overtake them. Do you think a brash and arrogant leader like Nicolas Sarkozy – whose disgusting election campaign involved him being portrayed as a disco dancer – wants to be faced with such a state?'

French Aspergistan movement supporters have been subject to long campaigns of harassment, since political parties advocating religion are banned and the constitution of the state of Aspergistan is seen as subversive.

Archived message from court records: Our appointed defence lawyer informed the Paris Delegation that this statement was unhelpful to their defence.

'We were the Jacobins of the Shy people. Robespierre's beheadings were to stop people from talking. The ballrooms and masquerades of the aristocracy – they could no longer be tolerated. Marie Antoinette: what is she a prototype of? Marie Antoinette is the ultimate Extrovert-Supremacist. Before her beheading, her hair was cut off and she was driven through Paris in an open cart, wearing a plain white dress. It was known that her era would end. Look at these vulgar leaders like Nicolas Sarkozy and Carla Bruni: they are part of her lineage. Do they represent us? How can any Shy Radical tolerate that? How can we be expected to assimilate in a state that votes for that? Cart and plain white dress for Carla Bruni too.'

LATIN AMERICA DELEGATION: SHY GUEVARA

HAVANA, CUBA: The Latin American delegation resolved to immediately halt the expansion of salsa, carnival, rumba and zumba activity as the sole form of foreign representation abroad.

LA PAZ, BOLIVIA: Shy Radicals archival historians have claimed Che Guevara as a proto-Shy Radical: 'In the iconic Che Guevara shot, you notice this: he is not making eye-contact. His eyes are somewhere between that look that Extroverts mistake for aloofness, Autistism, self-absorption, and dreaminess. He famously said: 'If you tremble with indignation at every injustice then you are a comrade of mine.' But ask yourself why people don't notice that word 'tremble' – which an Extrovert-normative reading of the text erases and thus subjugates his real politics.'

MOTION: The Fado delegation and Sevdah delegation are working hand in hand to address the problem.

WEST BENGAL BREAKAWAY DELEGATION

WEST BENGAL, INDIA: Threats to the state ceased to come from the Naxalite Maoist assaults on landlords. A new faction threatened to tear apart 'shining India'.

A militant faction started in the Tagore art school in Santiniketan (translated as 'abode of peace') in West Bengal. At first the faction practiced Japanese brush painting under a banana tree, in imitation of alumni Satyajit Ray. But this was not enough to preserve the wider culture. The faction sought to revive the Bengali film industry and overturn the domination of Bollywood. At first, it was thought by the government that this move was led by post-Partition refugees from Bangladesh, the former East Pakistan. It was thought this was Islamic fundamentalism – clamping down on a decadent, morally corrupt India. But this was something else. News is still coming in to this day.

QUEBEC BORDERS DELEGATION

Quebec, Canada: The Quiet Revolution was a period during the 1960s fathered by the Liberal politician Jean Lesage that saw a surge in Quebec nationalism and pride in Francophone identity, summed up by the electoral slogan Maîtres chez nous ('masters in our own home'). The period saw the establishment of universal health care and the nationalisation of key industries such as hydro-electric power which remain a source of pride to this day. It saw the dismemberment of the Roman Catholic Church and the disempowerment of nuns. But it was neither quiet nor a revolution. The business of politics and elections continued to be carried out via salesman slogans, and all power lay firmly in the hands of the Extrovert class.

The Quebec Borders delegation has sought to reclaim the slogan Maîtres chez nous and restore it to its true meaning. Lesage's other electoral slogan *L'équipe de tonnerre* ('the terrific team') remains distasteful to us.

Complaints amongst our Paris delegation and Quebec-Borders delegation mirror one another, with the same problems with discourse on banning introspective Muslim practices and identities, along with a threat to the right to anonymity.

CANADA AND AMERICA: Canada was a place where Shy Radicals sought refuge from the United States – a hideout. An extradition request remains outstanding on a number of delegates, resulting in an escape to Quebec.

Already, unlike its other Western Anglophone cousins Britain and Australia, Quebec has a thriving francophone twenty-four hour cafe culture in replacement of the 'pub' and binge culture in all its major cities. This has since been scapegoated by the Extrovert-class mass media as responsible for the separatist Shy Radicals state. A Shy Radical delegation has broken out on the borders of the Quebec struggle...

PAN-AFRICANIST BREAKAWAY DELEGATIONS

ALGIERS, ALGERIA: After the war of Independence, Algiers had become a Mecca for revolutionary movements in 1970s - seen as the nation that fought the enslaver and won. Algiers was the central node for transnational resistance: insurgents from then Rhodesia, Vietnam, Colombia, Germany, Portuguese Africa and other areas where armed groups sought refuge and hospitality.

Former colonial mansions and colonial beaches were opened up to them as a base of operation. The Black Panthers had several Field Marshals in exile there – seeking to build symbolic and strategic solidarity between Third World Liberation movements and First World oppressed minorities in the belly of the beast.

The opening of this relationship was consolidated by the first festival of Pan-Africanism in 1969 held in the revolutionary capital. This monumental event was documented by William Klein in the film essay *Festival panafricain d'Alger*. Jazz saxophonist Archie Shepp and Miriam Makeba took centre-stage in this cultural exchange. The film was not endorsed at the Introfada that year the elevation of compulsive drumming rhythms, men on horses with macho ceremonial rifle shots. howling in the street, masked flamboyance. The 2nd Pan-African Festival was held in 2009, adopting the language of 'diversity'. The Shy Radicals delegation has decided unanimously to boycott this festival until it recognises an Africa beyond extrovert-normative Africa.

The Black Panthers in exile soon left the country due to the Algerian desire to form diplomatic relations with the American embassy, damaged after several plane hijackings. Eldridge Cleaver, author of memoir *Soul on Ice,* notoriously, went on to become a born-again Christian and support Richard Nixon. However, five remain as the Shy Five, after an African Safari hunt, where the animals were impossible to find: the meerkat, the aardvark, the porcupine, the aardwolf, the bat-eared fox. In contrast to the Big Five - the game-hunter trophies: the African lion, African elephant, Cape buffalo, African leopard, and rhinoceros - these animals were nocturnal, elusive, impossible to find by Safari hunter. The aardvark even worked to burrow holes and tunnels for the rest of the Shy Five to hide. Hence the remaining Black Panthers, formed units and cells: the Black Meerkat, the Black Aardvark, the Black porcupine, the Black Aardwolf, the Black bat-eared fox to form a break-away movement for the continent, so we could operate as a base operation against the Extrovert World Order.

TRIPOLI, LIBYA: We have received breaking news that the Pan-Africanist delegation has ceased their support for Colonel Gaddafi against the NATO aggression and occupation.

WikiLeaks disclosures revealed that Saif al-Islam Gaddafi and other family members had used over $1 million of state treasure for a private New Year's party featuring performances from Beyoncé and Mariah Carey. On hearing the news, the Shy Radical delegation immediately dropped their support and ceased any diplomatic ties between the two factions. Gaddafi, with his flamboyant costumes, has violated our limits: he is an Extrovert-Supremacist leader.

NOTTING HILL CARNIVAL – TOTAL EXTROVERT-SUPREMACISM

LONDON, ENGLAND: Notting Hill Carnival was sold in the post-imperial British state as the epitome of the vibrant contented urban citizenry. As the festival became more established, leaders of the Conservative Party took advantage of photo opportunities at the festival, with Conservative opposition leader William Hague drinking from a coconut in a rolled-up denim shirt being the quintessential image.

Originally, Notting Hill Carnival was billed as a festival of the oppressed. Claudia Jones, the pioneer of intersectional analysis, known as the 'mother of Notting Hill Carnival', sowed its roots into British cultural life. The festival has been running since 1966 and has grown into Europe's largest street festival, attracting millions of people over a Bank Holiday weekend in August. Many of our Shy and Introvert people have experienced the festival as an assault and an onslaught.

The Caribbean notion of 'mas', which defined the politically subversive nature of the festival, traces its roots to the *carnevali* held before Lent in Italy, which were in turn taken by French plantation owners in the 1780s to the West Indies. Slaves mimicked – or mocked – the masked balls, adding their own African influences and Indian fabrics to the mix. The first carnival proper was held in Trinidad in 1833 (although this date is disputed; some say 1834, others 1838) to mark the end of slavery in the Caribbean, and Caribbean carnivals now take place around the world.

But were these rebellious historical roots acknowledged by the drunken crowds? There is a parade of headdresses, sequins, feathers, a kaleidoscope of loud colours. There is penetrative noise and coercive feel-good vibes that many of our people are familiar with. This time it only intensified. This is described as 'energy' and 'spirit'. But we are left feeling drained, not energised. We see the men pissing in the streets and we see total surface, not spirit. Jovial conformity, not free-spirited resistance.

Finally, finally, after the Introfada Spring, as a matter of public amnesty and relief, there came men who in full authentic freedom could honestly say just how much they hated the festival...

Extrovert-Supremacism out of Africa...
Extrovert-Supremacism out of Asia...
Extrovert-Supremacism out of the Americas...
Extrovert-Supremacism out of the Middle East...
Extrovert-Supremacism out of the Ghetto...

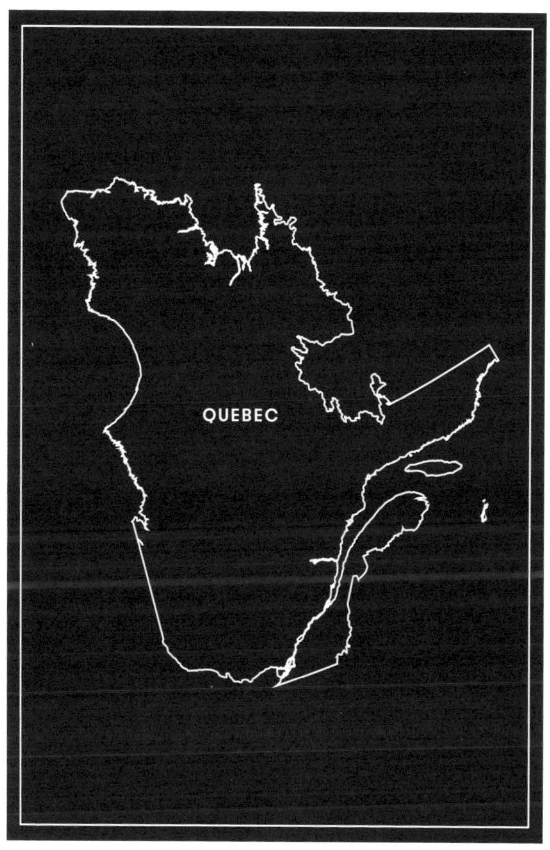

Quebec, Canada

ELEVEN

ALLIES AND COALITION PARTNERS IN THE INTROFADA

It was once believed that categories of oppressed people could only express liberation through speaking up: act up, raised fists, perched on soap boxes, megaphones, assertive slogans, street parades, occupying public space. Loud PRIDE; not humble pride: humility and modesty were to be buried alive in the name of some perpetually deferred, progressive goal. Have you ever heard collaborators with the oppressor-class say: *Yes, I am an extrovert-supremacist because I am a Black woman?* A Malcolm X social media relays a quote 'So early in my life, I learnt that if you want something, you had better make some noise'. In reality, this means accepting the existence of the order in its original stratified form: a hurdle to overcome, a higher authority to speak above, a perch to shout to, a rung up the ladder. Do we reinforce or break the existing order of things? 'Make some noise' became a catcall of the Superstar Trendy Club DJ in a way the young black revolutionary couldn't foresee – co-opted into the system. Therefore, true liberation for all humanity exists when we acknowledge that there is no need for a raised voice, when at last we can all be Shy and quiet until the end of history.

There are other political movements who recognise this fact of life and world history, and are prepared to move against the power structure. It is part of our vital work as a vanguard force to direct these movements as a united front. Toward the path of true Liberation.

THE QUIET GARDEN MOVEMENT

Come with me by yourselves to a quiet place and get some rest...

– **Mark, 6:31**

The Quiet Garden Movement was originally set up in the 1990s, in the Golden Age of the Sensitive White Man, by an Anglican priest; a global Internationalist movement of three hundred quiet gardens, parks and rural settings, operating like autonomous cells, for the purposes of spiritual rejuvenation. Whilst many in the movement must live in the heart of congested urbanity, often nothing can be heard in these quiet gardens apart from the chirping of birds. Speaking for the London Telegraph, our ally Reverend Roderick says: 'The Quiet Garden Movement is about giving people permission to step back and experience a sense of stillness and wonderment... We have all become so hyperactive, and our lives so subsumed in cacophony that we cannot hear the sound of a falling flower in a quiet garden.'

These gardens open up the private landlord-or family-owned space into communal space through joint ownership of the means of contemplation. It is hoped that they may offer a space away from that of the noisy and congested after-work pub or bar. The model offers an alternative to that of the high-street chain store or fast-food franchise. Quiet gardens have also been set up in South Yorkshire by a prisoners' group working with a church by the reclamation and transformation of derelict land.

Zones of tranquillity were often licenced and contained. How were they to be truly protected by the citizenry? Did they influence local council and government policy? Could they be bought out, developed? Could they resist the imperial growth of the high street?

During the London riots, keepers of the quiet gardens suggested they act as points of escape after the looting and destruction of several high-street shops. The Shy Radicals movement is in negotiation on how the two tendencies of the rioter and the gardener can work in mutual partnership – as hammer and sickle, rather than gardener being picket fence to keep the rioter out.

THE GAY SHAME MOVEMENT

> *'Out of the closets...'*
> *'Come out... '*

The two slogans of the Gay Pride movement can not be readily used as point of call out for Introvert emancipation. Why is it that extrovert-normativity is seen as the final point of Liberation? Corporate Pride street celebrations with ostentatious floats all seen as the endpoint of a triumphant world order. The mainstream became embedded into us by figures such as prime-time chat show hosts on a perpetual performance wheel. This is not the way we measure progress. All roads do not lead to the mainstream.

The Gay Shame Movement began life in Brooklyn, New York towards the close of the 1990s, when the ascendency of alternative subcultures into the mainstream was on the wane. The movement formed as a resistance to the mainstreaming and corporate domination of PRIDE street parades globally. Offshoot events such as the Annual Festival of Homosexual Misery in London also sprang up. The LGBTQI-led movement acknowledged the co-option of Gay Liberation into commercialisation, de-politicisation and corporatisation. Their San Francisco chapter put it thus: 'With corporate sponsors such as American Express, Bank of America, US Bank, Wells Fargo, AT&T, Comcast, Macy's, Bechtel, Clorox, Lennar and Morgan Stanley, the current agenda for the Center is one of cold, consumeristic capitalism. Instead of being a Robin Hood-esque pipeline that feeds cash into programs that actually serve the community as a whole, the Center invests their corporate largesse into creating and nourishing a queer consumer/entrepreneur culture.' In the 1990s, the queer subcultures that made up the zine fairs and the underground handmade small-press publications merged together. At earlier stages, when introverts were bullied at school, the Shy and quiet children were often taunted with the word 'gay' (as documented by our student movement). The DIY aesthetics continued within the agitprop of the movement. The movement also incorporated a resistance to Capitalist state legitimation. At first, this took the form of a counter-attack on the notion of gay marriage, and later included an overlapping concern with prison abolition and gentrification. Gay Shame chose Tire Beach as one of the sites of their counter-festival, a rotting industrial park on the San Francisco Bay, where discarded MUNI streetcars are dumped and a concrete factory borders a small grassy area. A vital principle of the group's argument against neoliberalism lies in the access and 'freedom' of public space versus the privatization and gentrification of space.

The concept of national borders was also resisted, building solidarity with LGBTQI asylum claimers, who were victims of detention centre and abusive Home Office policies. The movement continues to use the hashtag #GayShame, which has been intertwined with the tweets of Shy Radicals activists during phases of the Introfada. During the Notting Hill Introfada, they adopted the Shy Radicals Film training programme and the movement had each other's back.

THE QUAKERS

Messages of solidarity have been sent by the international Quaker movement, now a coalition partner of the Shy Radicals movement. Quaker groups have been holding silent vigils outside the prison cells of Shy Radicals political prisoners and are attending their court appearances.

In a core text of the Introvert Studies programme *Let Your Words be Few: symbolism of speaking and silence among seventeenth-century Quakers* Richard Bauman teaches us that this solidarity has its roots in the very inception of the Quakers movement: 'Part of the Quakers' understanding of the efficacy of the spiritual ministry rested on their theory of communication and rhetorical power. They believed that spiritual truth of a religious message stemmed from its source, God speaking within. Because the Inward Light was everywhere unitary and identical, true communication and persuasion were effected by the reaching of the Light in another person. Truth was felt in the resonant chord struck within one's conscience by another's message.'

Within you there is a stillness and sanctuary that you can retreat to anytime. Read the invitation to drop-in silence at a Friends House.

SAVE OUR LOCAL LIBRARY CAMPAIGNS

Potential for recruitment… Potential for raising consciousness of the bigger picture. Every town is fertile territory. As a strategy, if a library is threatened with closure, organise the local demographic to take out every single book in the library's catalogue, just so that we are clear as to whom the institution really belongs.

OTAKU SUBCULTURES

The *otaku* subculture (a term mistranslated in Western Extrovert-Supremacist terminology discourse as 'geek') flourished in post-war Japan, characterised by so-called obsessive collecting of fan memorabilia relating to anime and manga. We wondered what the possibilities of a subculture were when it was not attached to insatiable consumption. What was *otaku* without capitalism?

1989 saw the persecution of all Shy, Introvert and Autistic Spectrum peoples in Japan. This was the year of the *otaku* serial killer. Rapid stigmatisation followed the case of Tsutomu Miyazaki, the '*Otaku* Murderer'. This series of murders was carried out by an obsessive fan of several young girls using scenarios drawn from manga comics. It resulted in the scapegoating of all of us. The government also needed to be seen to be doing something and exploited the populist fearmongering. The '*Otaku* Murderer' case gave a negative connotation to fandom from which it has not fully recovered. The usage of '*otaku*', however, is used for teasing or self-deprecation, but the unqualified term remains negative. The identification of *otaku* turned negative again in late 2004 when Kaoru Kobayashi kidnapped, sexually assaulted and murdered a seven-year-old first-grade student. Japanese journalist Akihiro Ōtani speculated that Kobayashi's crime was committed by a member of *figyua moe zoku* ('figurine-lover gang') subculture even before his arrest. Although Kobayashi was not an *otaku*, the degree of social hostility against *otaku* increased. *Otaku* were seen by law enforcement as possible suspects for sex crimes, and local governments called for stricter laws controlling the depiction of eroticism in *otaku* materials.

A small delegation of the *otaku* subculture travelled especially to North Korea in search of a missing limited edition of a comic. The author was rumoured to be living in Pyongyang. In a letter home to their families, they said they had found sanctuary in North Korea away from the pressures and expectations of consumer-capitalism.

YAMABUSHI DELEGATION

The *Yamabushi* predate the Shy Radical movement. It started with the ascetic mountain hermits of Japan with their special conch shells, accorded with special, some say magical, powers.

The *Yamabito* are mountain people in the folk tales in prehistoric Japan, often depicted in pottery, monuments and oral history. The Introvert Studies programme established at School of Oriental and African studies (University of London) has a number of PHD research programmes led by the Yamabushi delegation in order to reclaim our heritage.

NIQABIS

Years earlier, Shy Radicals had sent a message of diplomatic solidarity to those affected by the niqab ban – and these individuals were sought as coalition partners in the Internationalist Shyria Law summit. We warned that this would signal a threat to the right to anonymity in public space in the future. In addition, we objected to the discourse, which was in all cases limited to an Extrovert-normative reading of the women's intentions. Hence no aspect of the commentariat discussed the women's inward journey, in relation to an investigative history of the prophets, or Muhammad's wives and companions. It was seen only as an antagonistic gesture – an f—you to French Liberal society, for example. Or in other cases as covering the non-existent scars and wounds of domestic violence: it was assumed that women who wore the face veil were always submissive, subjugated and oppressed. But this is the way the Extrovert-Supremacist pig views us Shy peoples too. In this discourse, the limits of the Extrovert-Supremacist imagination were exposed.

TWELVE

DIRECTORY OF HELPFUL SERVICES:
DIAL 0-0-1...
INTROVERT EMERGENCY
RESCUE HOTLINE

Adding to the list of existing emergency state-funded services - the police, the ambulance and fire brigade - the Introvert Rights Association pushed for a trial national service of the Introvert Emergency Rescue Hotline.

'I wish I hadn't gone [to that party] last night! I should have gone with my instincts and gone home, which is what I wanted to do... I stood on my own in a corner of the room most of the time, not knowing what to do.'

Automated reply: *Next time. Dial 0-0-1... your Introvert Emergency Rescue Hotline. Your right to be alone.*

Drivers were provided for anyone seeking rescue. Black cars fitted with specially black-tinted windows. A hotline was fitted for anyone seeking an excuse to leave an unwanted social relationship. First aid kits were provided with users registered given their favourite tea bag, a zipped black hoodie, comfort blanket and selection of used books (donated by charities). In extreme situations of company confinement, a professionally designed rescue operation consisting of temporary sensory deprivation, kidnapping and hooding was provided.

Full training was provided to all staff. A vocational diploma was established by several adult colleges and further education institutions. There was disquiet and concern about whether a staff simply trained in introvert issues could be considered to provide a genuine peer service. Concern was expressed as to whether discrimination and deliberate neglect by an extrovert-oriented staff, who did not treat the complaints with sufficient weight, would arise. Additional concern was expressed as to whether the service was independent of the state.

The switchboard was frequently jammed. The service doubled and tripled from its original purpose as a rescue service. It was also used as a post-trauma counselling service. Patrols of the Introvert Emergency hotline also travelled around cities at night – helping those stranded or who felt alienated at night. The hotline often ran into conflict with other emergency services: operating at odds with ambulance and police services use of sirens, cordons and alert signals. The Vegas Foundation also issued a number of press releases suggesting the service created new barriers to integration. At periods during Christmas and New Year's Eve, the service was stretched beyond its resources – leading to its eventual dismantlement.

Discontinued by the state and local councils, the initiative made significant progress in raising awareness of a new anti-social phenomenon. The final closure of the emergency line came during the period of the annual Eurovision song contest where an operating member of staff engaged in a criminal operation to shut down the contest. At trial, the aider plead guilty citing it was in 'aid of my people'. The archive material for this short-lived public service remains, housed in the Bishopsgate Institute in London.

ARCHIVED MESSAGE FOR TRAINING PURPOSES:

Operator: *Caller, I will put you on hold.*

Caller: *I want to disappear...*

Operator: *You have a right to walk away.*

Operator: *This call was recorded for training purposes. I will divert you to an aider.*

Caller: *The train carriage home is getting rowdy... It's reaching a level I can no longer tolerate... I think it is a lads' night out or something, or a stag do... I need another carriage. I went to the quiet coach. But people are talking there. Can you be quiet please? They laughed at me. I need quiet police... I can't get out.*

Aider: *Stay calm.*

Caller: *Their laughing is getting louder.*

Aider: *We will be on our way shortly.*

Caller: *I am hurting here...*

Aider: *First Aid Kits will be provided. Any sensory overload...*

Caller: *Yes, it's too much.*

Aider: *The hood and goggles will be provided. We will be with you shortly. Hold on.*

TRAINING ARCHIVE SELECTION:

Dial 0-0-1...

I am here in the local library to study. I witnessed even the librarians chatting... Who can I report to? I mean, this is supposed to be one of the few protected public spaces for citizens – an oasis in a land of consumption. Where else can we be like this? What are my rights? The librarians were doing nothing about it. They were even joining in with the banter. So, what higher authority could I turn to?

Dial 0-0-1...

The new workplace... The management forced me to attend the office Christmas party. I can't hide behind the photocopier. I am here now... I made a mistake.

Dial 0-0-1...

> *I thought this small island off the coast of Greece was where I could make archaeological discoveries. When I saw the litter of beer cans... The island was supposed to be my break and my escape.*

SCRAPPED ARCHIVED ADVERTISING SLOGAN:

> *Until the transformation comes, we are here to act as Samaritans.*
>
> *It was suggested at the time that expressing such views may harm the organisations grants and funding.*

While the service no longer remained, the demand for the service would not go away. Former users, and those in need, are still dialling 0-0-1 to this day.

AXIS OF RESISTANCE
OF THE WHITE MAN

'We are all Sensitive White Men'

– Shy Radical slogan

The Sensitive White Man is an oppressed class.

The cosy antiquarian second-hand bookshop is not the oppressor. The loss-making small press, producing delicate handmade editions, is not the Enemy. Every bastion of the Sensitive White Man is vulnerable. This requires our intervention.

The interior life of Van Gogh in his bedroom, in his starry night, in his diaries, paintings and letters, in the corner of a cafe or billiard room, in the sanatorium. He is a figure from history to whom we can relate. The Shy Radical movement resolves to stand, in full shoulder-to-shoulder solidarity, with the Sensitive White Man through his darkest moments. We realign ourselves internally and internationally. He belongs in the camp of the oppressed. We are at one with his sensibilities. He does not need to 'man up'. We recognise the grievances and frustrations of the inner-city Sensitive White Man.

Shy Radicals seeks a fundamental subversion of all conventions for identifying privilege. In reconstructing histories of the universal, the figure of the Sensitive White Man in history must be salvaged and separated from the figure of the Great White Man. What is chauvinism but Extrovert-Supremacism in its reduced masculine form? The weary eyes of a Rembrandt burning into his chiaroscuro self-portraits... These are figures from history who we wish to reclaim, rather than usurp.

What is the shape of privilege? Shy Radicals is not just about revolutionary empowerment and defence strategy for the Shy peoples, but a revolutionary remapping of the totem of identity politics. Do not assume a vertical axis of stratification, with cultural elitism and privilege at the top. The levels of class and power do not begin from the ground up. The lowly are not at the bottom of the heap. Our radical imagination digs into the soil... It is underground, from the rich organic life downwards to forgotten treasure, layers of a thousand lives, coal, fuel, mineral resources, archaeological treasure, the rich life of the earth.

THE CORPORATE GHETTO: BLACK EXTROVERT-SUPREMACISM

Now compare the poverty of the Sensitive White Man to corporate Afro-America. Take your pick of any generic corporate rap and R'N'B star: Pharell's 'Happy', Beyonce's 'Crazy', 50 Cent's 'Candy Shop'... These figures embody and export power in the Extrovert World Order. They embody capital and visibility, but not necessarily Black Power. Their 'success' depends on supplying a warm opiate. Everything feels good. Black Extrovert-Supremacism is streamlined into the Extrovert-Imperialist arsenal.

Go further into the Sensitive White Man's world... The world of page poetry, the small press, the poetry magazine, all totally within the Sensitive White Man's domain. Yet this world captures his present plight. No matter how many prizes a page poem wins, the crowds never expand much beyond the intimate. It is inherent to the very form of page poetry that it resists the mass crowd, no matter how much state funding it is offered. There is no stadium tour for the page poet. Social capital is not the goal of the poetry gathering.

Then there are the hands-in-the-air-and-in-your-face genres of performance poetry, spoken word, Def Jam slam poetry. Stars from such genres will for the purposes of their credibility distance themselves from the canon of the Sensitive White Man. The Extrovert street does not respect our ways. I don't read Keats cos I am from da streets, voices a high macho spoken word artist. The Shy Radical bedroom treasures the Keats cottage. The Shy Radical reads beside the omnipresent log-fire.

Think of a lo-fi indie label, a folk singer in a cardigan, avant-garde noise recordings only distributed in small-edition zines, all on the verge of disappearing. Think of a fringe theatre producing handmade marionette puppet theatre on a boat, barely surviving on its local authority grant, versus a high-street musical production of the gospel Hollywood blockbuster *Sister Act.*

It is not clear which is marginal, underappreciated, in need of our support? Is it not clear who is the oppressor and who is the oppressed? Who is really the voice of the margins? Who is powerful and who is powerless? Who is the flea and who is the fat cat? Let the Sensitive White Man join us in the struggle – our liberation is bound up together. The Shy Radical Internationalist movement vows to liberate the Sensitive White Man.

UNESCO YEAR OF CULTURAL APPRECIATION OF THE SENSITIVE WHITE MAN

The Sensitive White Man has a universal gift for humanity. His cultural talent for singing of angst, depression, melancholia and woe is universally appreciated across people and borders. Even groups amongst the marginalised and subaltern relate to him. Hence we see the Morrissey and Smiths fans in the Latino slums and ghettoes of Los Angeles. Listen to the pain of Kurt Cobain, the glacial bleakness of Ian Curtis, the fragility of Elliott Smith between the acoustic strums, the erudite isolation of the Manic Street Preachers' Richey Edwards, the depressive witticisms of Leonard Cohen. Even in genres such as black metal is to be found an articulation of this depressive under-blanket in a thick form. We have to reach the conclusion that no one does this better. This is the authentic realm of mastery of the Sensitive White Man.

THE 1990S: THE SEATTLE INTROFADA

In the Western world, the 1990s is a period our ministry of culture has deemed the Golden Age of the Sensitive White Man. The decade began with Tim Burton's film *Edward Scissorhands*, with Edward becoming a romantic icon for the movement. This was Introvert man in all his misunderstood, gifted beauty, in an ugly Day-Glo world, on the big screen.

Simultaneously, in the urban centres of the West during the

1990s marginalised people of colour produced new genres of music in the opposite direction. We saw this in the bling-bling of gangsta rap: bouncing Cadillacs, designer brand names and Gucci time. Then, an acceleration of tempos in genres such as jungle, drum'n'bass, speed garage. The Asian Underground formed a hybrid of breakbeats mixed with Bollywood anthem samples.

Sonic the Hedgehog – a blue hedgehog running at superfast speeds – was born as the mascot of the computer game company Sega, then at the peak of its popularity. The computer game continued to develop these trends with the marketing of the Sony PlayStation: the flagship game Wipeout introducing rave tracks into a futuristic high-speed racing game. This was no longer the world of the bedroom programmer and the Dungeons & Dragons enthusiast. The world of computer games sought to be fashionable and cool – and ultimately part of Trendy Club.

The 1990s also saw the expansion of the mega-club brand, with superstar DJs becoming global household names. It was now obligatory to go to Trendy Club whether you enjoyed it or not. The Sensitive White Man provided us with a sanctuary in their midst – we sought asylum in his words and records.

This was the year that the underground alternative rock sound of 1990s grunge music from Seattle and beyond became globalised on MTV music networks: Nirvana, Alice in Chains, R.E.M. brought the sensibility of the Great American Sensitive White Man overground to new commercial mainstream peaks, and reminded the world that 'Everyone hurts… Hold on'. Nice guys finished first.

This trend trickled into Europe. The European sounds of the Sensitive White Man include England's Radiohead and the fragile hushed strums of Scotland's Belle and Sebastian at their peak. Smashing Pumpkins remained in depressive mode and had not yet turned into the poppy, cheery and melodic Zwan. More underground, the delicate, austere sound of slowcore lo-fi bands such as Low and Codeine slowed the rock tempo to a sunken heartbeat. Voices of desolation and fragility that only the ethnic cultures of the white middle classes could produce. But they spoke for all of us. Shy and Introvert people from all over the world related to the tragic plight of the Sensitive White Man, this delicate and tragic figure.

The risk was always that the Shy peoples would be absorbed into the Extrovert-Supremacist economy. The so-called 'Studio Introvert' rather than an authentic Real Introvert.

Shyness and so-called social awkwardness would become hollowed out into a fashion item. Although deep down some of us admit a perverse enjoyment in seeing the LIE (Liberal Intoxicated Extrovert) people try so hard to look like us, embracing so-called goth and grunge style on the catwalk and in fashion marketing.

All this was, at any rate, swiftly followed by a backlash in popular culture in Britain with lad culture – in the magazines Loaded and *FHM*, and later *Nuts* and *Zoo*. A mixture of glossy hyper-consumerist magazine content, sports interest, formatted soft pornography and Trendy Club ethos defining masculinity in the mainstream. The formula of *FHM* magazine was exported to growth Asian economies, with the largest circulations in India and the Philippines. In the world of music, laddism in the form of Oasis and retro-hedonism became the vogue. Again, these trends were exported to growing Eastern markets in South Korea and Taiwan. This expansion continues. The pain of earlier styles of authentic depressives turned into corporate emo for later generations, robbed of all authenticity.

The 1990s was too much for some. The rock icon Kurt Cobain committed suicide in 1994, and defined the era. The lyricist Richey James Edward went missing at the Severn Bridge... he is now declared officially dead.

In developed industrial nations, a high suicide rate still exists. Consider that of the more than 6,000 suicides that take place in the *UK* annually each year, 4,500 are men, mostly white men. Sensitive White Men. Suicide is now established as the biggest killer of young and middle-aged men. This phenomenon has been blamed on so-called 'man up' culture: a prevalent macho attitude that stops men from talking about their vulnerabilities and feelings, or derides them as effeminate for doing so. Perhaps the real reason men feel unable to speak openly and honestly of negative emotions is not so much because of masculine culture but Extrovert-Supremacist culture?

So consider, if Sylvia Plath is claimed by the college feminist movement as a victim of a patriarchal society, then what to read into these men who form the bulk of suicide cases? Our movement should claim them as the first Shy Radicals martyrs. From Nick Drake's whispers of despair to Aaron Schwartz's mark on cyberspace. All of them died for a greater cause. Shy Shaheed.

Shy Radicals unanimously resolves to push for the Internationalist demand for the UNESCO Year of Cultural Appreciation of the Sensitive White Man, when accorded a seat in the United Nations as Aspergistan.

FOURTEEN

VANGUARD MELANCHOLIA:
BLACK–BLACK POWER

Our task is to transform sorrow into strength.

– Chairman Mao

I wear black on the outside
'Cause black is how I feel on the inside...

– The Smiths, 'Unloveable' from *The World Won't Listen*

Little by little you know
We got the power
And the knowledge to move 'em
And still rock
A super song for the cause so
Feel the load on your brain for the episode
And we just begun, it's number one y'all
Brother Black, the B is back

– Public Enemy, 'B Side Wins Again' from
   Fear of a Black Planet

The Extrovert-Supremacist system teaches us that negative thinking is the source of all the world's problems. Negatives are to be eradicated. Happy Meals equal 'health'. Extrovert Supremacism always maintains its hegemony through a full spectrum of 'positivity'. From the 'Have a nice day, y'all' of the McJob workplace to its corporate colour scheme: bright reds and yellows. Negative-thinkers are the enemy within. An attitude that the system can't quite absorb.

We should note a famous prison conversation between Malcolm x and a fellow inmate that marked a step in the journey of the political awakening of the young revolutionary. In a prison cell, his cellmate outlines the mapping of references and associations of the word 'black' in popular usage. He follows the familiar critique of patterns of language where all 'black' things are associated with all things evil and undesirable, as a symptom of a White-Supremacist society. Black as evil. Black as doom. Black as negative.

Charles: *As soon as we get settled, we'll build you a darkroom in the basement, okay?*

Lydia: *My whole life is a darkroom. One big darkroom.*

– From the film *Beetlejuice*

What is the deeper reality of the situation? It is not just that Blackness is disdained at the level of appearance. This is an Extrovert-normative reading of events. Black is also the mood and disengaged world that this word connotes. It is more the case that the turn inwards – so-called black moods – are not valued in an Extrovert-Supremacist society. A black day. A black heart. Black bile.

When placed in company, dare we dwell within ourselves rather than chatter, thereby violating the sanctity of so-called social etiquette? Are we wet blankets? Are we misery guts? An Extrovert-Supremacist society will not tolerate our differences for all their claims of liberalism. We are not party to their party. Their Extrovert-Supremacist genres of music – such as turbo-folk, trance club music and funky house – do not allow time and space for any dissident mode of being. Just a total onslaught of positivity in the form of an assault of incessant repetitive beats. The big boom trucks of Notting Hill Carnival are the same, the experience of which has been documented in our Crisis Voices oral history project. What is called a 'commercial radio' station will iron out every vocal range and instrument into congenial Extrovert-blandness. Sensitivity and intelligence must be wiped out too. This is tyranny of smiley, positivist, Wahhabi Extrovert-Supremacism. And it something that must be brought to an end. We revolt, simply because we can no longer breathe.

In the classroom, in the playground, from teacher to pupil, in the lounge, into the workplace, from college to college, manager to worker.

Everyday Extrovert-Supremacism.

DAILY INTERROGATIONS:

Why are you being so miserable?
Don't you realise you are spoiling it for all of us?
Don't you speak?
Don't you smile?
Do you think you are above everyone?

The Extrovert class will take our way of being for aloofness, dumbness or stuck-up-ness.

What is 'miserabilism' in their world is an act of dissent for our peoples, living under a system that negates us. Figures like Wednesday Addams with her morbid humour emerge as heroic.

Consider the historical shift from melancholia to clinical depression. Melancholia is a form of fruitful dwelling – a retreat into a cave – something nourishing and rich. As the Socialist Patients' Collective puts it: 'To be healthy thus means to be expropriated and exploitable *[ausbeutbar zu sein]*.'

'If a worker nowadays visits his doctor and talks to him about a lot of symptoms (for example feelings of nausea, headache, dizziness, etc.) then the doctor does all he can to isolate those symptoms from their historic and biographic connections. He measures blood pressure, heartbeat and finally diagnoses some vegetative *Dystonie* ['disturbance of the autonomic neural system']; what about the relation with and the situation in the workplace and in the family home? There will be no interest, except as a side issue. Treatment as a business of exchange [*Tausheschaft*]: the symptoms have to be rigged up in such a way that they, as an economic demand [*Nachfrage*], will fit in with some supply [*Angebot*] of the medico-technical pharmaceutical industry, corresponding to each other.'

– Socialist Patients' Collective, *Turn Illness into a Weapon*

In 1980, social anxiety disorder was adopted by the DSM, the *Diagnostic and Statistical Manual of Mental Disorders*. The central principle of many therapy programmes indoctrinate patients into the idea of 'being positive'. This period also saw the expansion of the selective serotonin re-uptake inhibitors, with brand names such as Prozac and Paxil Extroverts, accompanied by advertisement campaigns featuring permanent plastic smiles. They will not tolerate your existence otherwise. There is no refuge or asylum in their world. The Extrovert class has a low tolerance threshold when it comes to negative emotions. There is no yin and yang. There is no co-existence. There is only negation and exile.

THE SOLUTION: THE BLACK POWER–SENSITIVE WHITE MAN ALLIANCE; OR, TOWARDS BLACK–BLACK POWER

As A. Sivanandan says, 'black is a political colour, not the colour of your skin... the colour of oppression today is black'.

Blackness must not be conflated with the technocratic managerial trend of 'diversity'. Black politics in the British context, that of a union of anti-imperialist peoples in the British context, a push towards power. This is how Black politics distinguished itself from later forms of 'diversity management', which did not seek to challenge the axis of power, the epistemology, the structure of stratification, but instead sought additive multicoloured foot soldiers.

To complete our task, we must combine two 1990s trends: gangsta rap, where we appreciate a certain subcultural mode of toughness (albeit a posture) in the face of an oppressive system, and the mode of the Sensitive White Man angst-ridden alternative rock musician under another oppressive system. To clarify our political stance: Gangsta rap cannot be accepted on its own terms.

Early generations of civil rights activists such as Delores Tucker and rappers such as Chuck D may object to the commodified bling lifestyle. No different from Turbo-folk, from the defeated Serbian nation/defeated Liberace/defeated Marie Antoinette fashion and hollowing of political substance to glittery lucrative self-parody. The message is absent.

Try this as an exercise. Rewatch the music video for two iconic mid-1990s hits: Eazy-E *Real Muthaphukkin' Gs* and Radiohead *Street Spirit (Fade Out)*. On the surface, the later seems to be a high art, melancholic black and white and acutely emotional (dare we say 'miserable') in stark contrast to the hyper-macho posturing gangsta video. Can we reflect and consider the two sensibilities – the hardened gangsta and the poetic depressive – being combined? Both reference the dimensions of 'street' knowledge. Both videos were shot in Los Angeles, produced in the aftermath of the 1992 Los Angeles riots triggered by Rodney King's police beating. Both feature barking guard dogs protecting territory. In the Radiohead video, singer Thom Yorke smashes a pane of glass in slow-motion. Both would be identified by extrovert society as a 'cause for concern'. We need the marriage of two alternate 'attitude problems'. We call this union *Black–Black Power*.

We propose a new union of these two modes of Blackness: that of the gloomy mood and depressive slumber, and that of the resistance of the former slave – let's call it Vanguard Melancholia. This is a reconstitution of an unjust order. The melancholia of Morrissey teamed with the wall-of-sound anger of Public Enemy, generating together. Behold the Fear of a Black–Black Planet. It will take a nation of millions to hold us back. Bury the Extrovert-Supremacists in our earth.

We need to protect our hood. But we need not Gs (gangstas) as a solution to our problems. But Sensitive Gs. That is to say sensitive introverts that you dare not fuck with.

FIFTEEN

COMPASS OF THE EXTROVERT CLASS: EIGHT EXTROVERT IDENTITIES

1 EXTROVERT-SUPREMACIST

Are you an Extrovert-Supremacist? Who maintains and advocates a clearly marked Extrovert-Supremacist society that preserves, names, and values Extrovert superiority?

2 EXTROVERT-VOYEURIST

Are you an Extrovert-Voyeurist? This means being an Extrovert Voyeur who would not challenge an Extrovert-Supremacist's stated beliefs. They desire quietness because it is interesting and pleasurable to them, and they seek to control the consumption and appropriation of quiet. They may express a fascination with culture, for example: consuming introvert culture without the burden of introvert life; consuming and appropriating introvert cultures, clothing, or spiritualities without the burden of Introvert hate and prejudice.

3 EXTROVERT-PRIVILEGE

Do you cling to your Extrovert-Privilege? An Extrovert Privileged person may critique extrovert-supremacy, but they maintain a deep investment in questions of 'fairness' and 'equality' that normalise extrovert-supremacy and extrovert rule. They may have a sworn goal of 'diversity'.

4 EXTROVERT-BENEFIT

Are you into Extrovert-Benefit? An Extrovert Benefit person is sympathetic to some aspects of shy radicalism, but only privately. They will not speak or act in solidarity in their networks, because they are benefiting through extrovert-supremacism in public.

5   EXTROVERT-CONFESSIONAL

Or is the Extrovert-Confessional your thing? An Extrovert Confessional person will speak about and point out extrovert-supremacy to some extent, but only as a way of being accountable to shy people after the fact. An Extrovert Confessional seeks validation from quiet, shy and autistic spectrum peoples.

6   EXTROVERT CRITICAL

Could you be an Extrovert-Critical? An Extrovert Critical person will take on board critiques of extrovert-supremacy and invest in exposing and marking the regime of extrovert-supremacy. They refuse to be complicit with the regime, and might be seen as extroverts speaking back to extroverts.

7   EXTROVERT TRAITOR

Are you an Extrovert-Traitor? An Extrovert Traitor actively refuses complicity in the regime of Extrovert-supremacy, names and speaks about what is going on, and intends to subvert extrovert authority and tell the truth at whatever cost.

8   EXTROVERT-ABOLITIONIST

And just how many Extrovert-Abolitionists are out there? An Extrovert-Abolitionist changes institutions that are historically based on extrovert rule, dismantles the system of extrovert-supremacy, and does not allow the regime or extrovert rule to reassert itself. No whoops, parties or trumpeting at the end to celebrate this, naturally.

SIXTEEN

THE DEMAND FOR REPARATIONS

Introverts don't 'move on'.

In solidarity with all global justice campaigns for historical recognition, from that of Columbus' invasion of America in 1492, to the return of the plundered Elgin Marbles and treasures of the Benin Kingdom from museum display cases, the ongoing Nakbah, and onward, the global Shy Radicals movement issues a universal resolution, from the bedroom, with our faces buried in our pillows, to say to the world at large:

'Don't move on.'

Take the long walk of Hillsborough – the death of ninety-six people at a football game, the largest police cover-up in European state history, in full compliance with an Extrovert-Supremacist media system, with government by distraction – only after twenty-seven years of struggle did the families achieve recognition of the truth, and justice in court. The former prime minister David Cameron echoing the corridors of power said – in a way demeaning to all introspective people – that the longing for truth was like 'a blind man, in a dark room, looking for a black cat that wasn't there'. Was it not to the benefit of the world that such people's struggle did not move on? From that moment of truth, all other retrospective justice campaigns can take inspiration. What festering darkness remains over those years was the pure blackness of truth. To not 'move on' is the true stuff of heroism. Let us forever brood in the dark room then. Close the curtains. Fester onwards...

Every broken soul demands justice, reconciliation, hope, parity and fairness. Don't move on. Moving on as representative of the continuation of life, moving on as the ultimate life ethic of the future, is the received morality of a shallow Extrovert-normative entertainment industry. Sitcoms, *Friends*, relationship dramas, κ-pop songs, cheap thrills, advertising fix-it slogans, rollercoaster rides, and so on. Think: these forms of 'entertainment' do not allow us the same slow pace and open space of the Ingmar Bergman film or the latest Iranian cinematic masterpiece. Reflection, maturation, distillation, marination: there is no fast-food justice system. To 'let go' is to comply with the corporative Godhead: laying off workers, government without accountability. Government by Shyria Law will not permit this.

Don't 'let go'.

1   FINANCIAL COMPENSATION FOR THE BILLIONS MADE THROUGH GLOBALISING OUR PAIN

The Extrovert World Order owes us. This compensation will be drawn from the pockets of those who have plundered our resources, disturbed our peace and dispossessed us.

The Extrovert World Order was erected on the backs of our peoples... Their entertainment industry made its billions through globalising our ridicule – an exported film and TV industry of media formats designed to keep us in our place. Teen drama movies that framed us as a perpetual underclass and figures of ridicule, forever expanding their markets into Asia and beyond.

It was said that Labour leader Ed Miliband lost the 2015 general election due to his resemblance to a 'nerd'. It was said that Donald Trump won the 2016 election due to being the high-school-corridor-jock-bully. Just think: your system affects us at the highest level of power. The Extrovert-normative mass media condemn 'loners' to a fate as instigators of deranged acts of terror and high-school mass shootings. We suffered the teen movie unto death...

The entire production process was built as a system of uneven development. It is only fair that the obscene inequality of star salaries that has been accumulated in the world of glossy images should be redistributed. This includes loss of earnings. Retrospectively, 'stars' of the Extrovert-Supremacist economy, from the socialite classes, from the fashion world to musicians, have behind the scenes a team of administrators and invisible production underclasses engaged in alienated labour. No more 'reality' TV to keep up with their self-appointed icons. Our reality will be fully recognised. The glittery, glossy and the glamorous…The Extrovert class possesses no right to rule. The Extrovert class has colonised our living rooms, with print and broadcast media parading their lifestyles. Divestment and sanctions on all celebrity capital.

Warning: we hold as a self-evident truth that all displays of luxury are the products of an Extrovert-Supremacist system. Private swimming pools and multi-storey buildings, brand-labelled handbags and footwear, their aspirational private planes and sports cars, ballrooms and so on. No more pool parties. Estates, holdings and mobile extravagances such as yachts and sports cars are not by any means safe. Our movement is licenced to seize and redistribute assets amongst our people. Their peoples' discomfort is a footstep in our journey of liberation.

This is retrospective economic justice. The survivors will govern and de-elevate the socialite-class positions of power, distribution, production and reproduction. The Extrovert class will cease to be an economic centre.

Compensation is just a small part of our demands.

2　**A FULL AND FORMAL APOLOGY MEANS RENUNCIATION OF FALSE AFFECTATION AND NICENESS**

The world will not sing in perfect harmony. Nothing will be solved by Extrovert people simply being 'alright'. 'How are you?', 'How was your weekend?' and other small-talk micro-aggressions will not be registered as real concerns anymore, until restitution.

A blacklist of public spaces where service staff have told our people to 'cheer up' will be drawn up in cooperation with the Enemy. Those cafes where we wished only to sit alone with black coffee and the company of a book. What else do you imagine a cafe is for? To establish profit and economic growth? We will seize every buck of every glossy cafe, and with that every chain bar, chain pub. We will return cafes to their original asocial social function for our people. Do not dare impose your feel-good ideology on us ever again.

3 REPATRIATION AND THE RETURN TO THE HOMELAND

Funds will be allocated toward establishing the Aspergistan state, sustaining our student bodies, universal pensions for the frail and elderly, underground networks, those who have suffered Introvert hate crime, and funding full-scale employment, arms and defence.

Citizens not accorded full Introvert rights are by natural right citizens of the Aspergistan state.

No amount of co-option into the system will appease us. The co-option of Introvert life into the studio. The 'studio Introvert': our styles of dress and life experiences by the 'alternative' indie music icons, independent cinema, the indie comic book and small-press poetry industry, will never heal this. This is mere social-democratic appeasement for the Introvert. Reform is not enough.

All profits from marine transportation, railways, highways, air travel, planes, parachutes and hot air balloons will be quietly redirected via natural right to return us to the prospective territories of the homeland state. These funds will be used to built a system of underground tunnels, vaults and catacombs to return us homeward.

We will only permit the future citizens of Aspergistan to travel home on the longest train journeys.

4 DEVELOPMENT AND REHABILITATION PROGRAMME

The painful memories of high school have not left us...

Our capacity for growth and development has been severely impaired since childhood, through our relationships with others, and throughout our student days. The boots were always firmly on our heads. Correctional compensation for damages are sought on behalf of all Shy, Introvert and Autistic Spectrum peoples. This extends to all of us as survivors, descendants, and victims of structural Extrovert oppression, the world over... Who can put a price on the emotional damage, permanent disadvantage and underdevelopment these institutions have exposed us to?

The Extrovert class could not tolerate our so-called 'reserved' natures. Starting from the classroom, into the office spaces, into the very structure and institutions of so-called representative democracy. Every hyped billboard in a public space as the Extrovert World Order plunders the Earth.

5 ECOLOGICAL JUSTICE

The synthetic will be totally abolished. The authentic will prevail.

We will create quiet parks, cosy indoor areas, fertile soils and fields. Flower shows in Extrovert-Supremacist nation states will feature education on the fertilising effects on compost. A state-funded tree-planting programme will cover all public fields – where raves and corporate festivals were held – returning them to the sacred woods, where constellations will be visible again, where the indigo of the night sky will be cherished by all.

We are with all victims of this violence. We do not stand alone. In the perverted cases of fur coats, leather jackets, the abuse wrought on animals; their inner worlds are trampled over in the name of showing-off. In the case of sports cars, and all luxury automobiles and transport, there is daily compulsion to display that chokes the environment. Audio-visual systems are not safe, as the vibrations of such system extend into spaces beyond their intended range. Now your people will be dependent on delineated permission by the Shy Radicals commissaries. Space and volume that have been violated in a previously tax-free oasis.

A halt has to be placed on the Extrovert-Supremacist system perpetuating itself. Our intervention is also for their own good, since their economy of emptiness, their engagement in such a system of display and competition is a landslide to headlong mutual self-destruction. We would be glad to see the destruction of their people and we desire to save the Earth and its resources from their thoughtless plunder.

We will create healing environments where birds can be heard to twitter, where the sound of the sea heals, where the full moon reflects perfectly on the river, where every citizen can dwell in caves and woods. All retrospective profits made by pharmaceutical industry on the multibillion industry antidepressants paroxetine, fluoxetine and related chemical fixes will taken reclaimed and redirected towards Aspergistan citizens. Aspergistani diplomatic representatives will work in cooperation with movement lawyers in all Extrovert nations to reclaim this money for its citizenry. We have every right to seize all assets underpinning the Extrovert-industrial complex.

6 THE ESTABLISHMENT OF PEACE

Closure. Closure after establishing total emancipation to establish pasture, to establish places where we can be quietly alone, drink a cup of tea, read books on a sofa and go for a gentle walk.

The entire process will be administered justly under the calculations of Shyria Law judicial system. This is the only assurance we are prepared to give. These are the only terms we will enter into a treaty of peace.

After the liberation, there will be no one to speak up to. True liberation will come when we can just stare at the ground and be our own autonomous political representatives. This is natural justice.

We are merely reclaiming what is ours: the right to life, space, quiet. We can then move forward and establish peace under the cool shade of the Aspergistan flag...

Full unconditional reparations for all Shy peoples, for the heroic sulkers, for the bullied and dominated, for the torn and humiliated. The first nations peoples of Aspergistan stand in solidarity with international calls for reparations for current and historical crimes, and demands recognition of the indignities we have suffered and puts forward the following six-point plan of action for reconciliation, reparation and justice. The popular girls may ignore us: but the demand for atonement festers on.

Draw the curtains. Don't let go...

The Shy Radical movement resolves: never get over it; get under it.

The world is our corner.

DONATE TOWARD THE FUTURE ASPERGISTAN STATE

ASPERGISTAN... THE UTOPIC HORIZON.

> **MERELY BY DESCRIBING YOURSELF AS A SHY RADICAL YOU HAVE STARTED ON A ROAD TOWARDS EMANCIPATION, YOU HAVE COMMITTED YOURSELF TO FIGHT AGAINST ALL FORCES THAT SEEK TO MAKE YOUR SHYNESS A STAMP THAT MARKS YOU OUT AS A SUBSERVIENT BEING.**
> **SHOW YOUR COMMITMENT.**

UNTIL THE FULL RECLAMATION OF REPARATIONS, WE NEED YOU TO SUSTAIN OUR CRUCIAL WORK.

CHIP IN TO CHIP AWAY: THE FOUNDATIONAL PILLARS OF ALL EXTROVERT-SUPREMACIST INSTITUTIONS WILL FALL.

SHY RADICALS ACCEPTS NO STATE OR CORPORATE FUNDING WHICH WOULD BE A MEANS TO SUBDUE AND COMPROMISE OUR VISION

1. NO CELEBRITY APPROVES OF THIS FUND ...
2. THIS IS FOR BLACK—BLACK POWER. FOR THE MELANCHOLIC DRIPS.
3. THERE WILL BE NO SMILING AFRICAN CHILDREN.
4. THIS IS FOR AGITATION. NO MORE LIVE AID, NO MORE CONCERT FOR BANGLADESH, NO MORE COMIC RELIEF.
5. WE WILL NOT ENDORSE UNDER ANY CIRCUMSTANCES FEEL - GOOD CHARITY GIVING.
6. NO 'OUTGOING' HIGH-STREET CHARITY MUGGERS PRETENDING TO CARE. NO COMPROMISE.
7. THERE WILL BE NO FIREWORKS.
8. THIS IS FOR THOSE WHO STRUGGLE UNDERGROUND.
9. THE SOLITARY ARE ALWAYS THE BEST REPRESENTATIVES OF SOLIDARITY.

SUPPORT US:

STANDING ORDERS CAN BE MADE TO:
BANK ACCOUNT: 00100100
SORT CODE: 01 01 01

DONATIONS CAN BE MADE ONLINE. CHEQUES CAN BE SENT, MADE PAYABLE TO SHY RADICALS. REPORTS OF OUR BANK ACCOUNTS BEING FROZEN REMAIN AN UNSUBSTANTIATED RUMOUR SPREAD BY THE VEGAS FOUNDATION.

£5 WILL PROVIDE ADVICE TO VICTIMS OF INTROVERT HATE CRIME AND DISCRIMINATION.

£10 WILL ALSO SUPPORT SOLIDARITY WORK WITH SHY RADICAL POLITICAL PRISONERS AND THEIR FAMILIES.

£20 WILL HELP BUILD OUR INTROFADA BASES AND SUPPORT INTROVERT SUPPORT WORK OVERSEAS.

£25 WILL HELP REHABILITATE THOSE SUBJECT TO COMPANY CONFINEMENT TORTURE REGIMES.

STANDING ORDERS AVAILABLE. ALL FUNDS ARE RECEIVED GRATEFULLY; EVEN IF IT IS JUST £1 A MONTH. CASH DONATIONS CAN ALSO BE SUBMITTED VIA RECORDED DELIVERY.

PLEASE FOLLOW LATEST PENDING NEWS AS INTROFADA STRUGGLES ARE PLANTED EVERYWHERE. FOLLOW @SHYRADICALS AND THE HASHTAG #INTROFADA ON TWITTER FOR LATEST UPDATES.

THIS IS FOR THE FINAL IRREVERSIBLE UNSETTLEMENT OF THE EXTROVERT WORLD ORDER. MAKE YOUR PRIVATE CONTRIBUTION TOWARDS BUILDING AN ALTERNATIVE. EXTROVERT-SUPREMACISM WILL BE ABOLISHED — SHY RADICALS PLEDGE TO THE FUTURE…THE WORLD IS OUR CORNER…

SHY RADICALS BY
Hamja Ahsan

This publication is published as part of Common Objectives, commissioned by Book Works from open submission and edited by Nina Power and Gavin Everall.

PUBLISHED AND DISTRIBUTED BY
Book Works

COMMISSIONING EDITOR
Nina Power

PROOFREADING BY
Jacob Blandy and Huw Lemmey

DESIGNED BY
Rose Nordin

PRINTED BY
Aldgate Press

Book Works receives National Portfolio funding from Arts Council England.

ISBN 978 1 906012 57 1

Book Works,
19 Holywell Row,
London EC2A 4JB
www.bookworks.org.uk

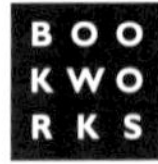

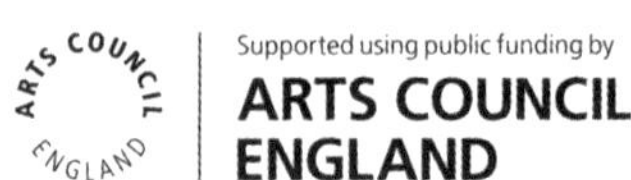

Common Objectives is a series of projects from artist/writer collectives or individual art practices engaged with emerging political struggles, rejecting the idea of culture as a playground for the elite, engaging in the potent mix of free discourse, solidarity and the production of new desires and prepared to break open old worlds, either in the virtual space of communication and networks, or in the concrete world of action, discourse and distribution.